214
Single Best Answer Questions
in
Gynaecology

with •Answers, •Explanations and •Basic Clinical Principles

for

Undergraduate and Postgraduate Students

214

Single Best Answer Questions

in

Gynaecology

With •Answers, •Explanations and •Basic Clinical Principles

for

Undergraduate and Postgraduate Students

Eranthi Samarakoon

MBBS, MS (Sri Lanka), FRCOG (UK)

Senior Lecturer and Head
Department of Obstetrics and Gynaecology
Faculty of Medicine, University of Peradeniya

Consultant Obstetrician and Gynaecologist
Teaching Hospital, Peradeniya, Sri Lanka

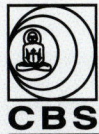

CBS

CBS Publishers & Distributors Pvt Ltd

New Delhi • Bengaluru • Chennai • Kochi • Kolkata • Lucknow • Mumbai
Hyderabad • Jharkhand • Nagpur • Patna • Pune • Uttarakhand

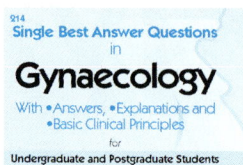

ISBN: 978-93-86310-61-3

Copyright © Author and Publisher

First Edition: 2017

Reprint: 2017, 2022

Published by Satish Kumar Jain and produced by Varun Jain for

CBS Publishers & Distributors Pvt Ltd

4819/XI Prahlad Street, 24 Ansari Road, Daryaganj, New Delhi 110 002, India
Ph: 011-23289259, 23266861, 23266867   Website: www.cbspd.com
Fax: 011-23243014   e-mail: delhi@cbspd.com; cbspubs@airtelmail.in
Corporate Office: 204 FIE, Industrial Area, Patparganj, Delhi 110 092

Ph: 011-4934 4934   Fax: 011-4934 4935   e-mail: publishing@cbspd.com;
                                               publicity@cbspd.com

Branches

• **Bengaluru:** Seema House 2975, 17th Cross, K.R. Road, Banasankari 2nd Stage, Bengaluru 560 070, Karnataka
  Ph: +91-80-26771678/79   Fax: +91-80-26771680   e-mail: bangalore@cbspd.com
• **Chennai:** 7, Subbaraya Street, Shenoy Nagar, Chennai 600 030, Tamil Nadu
  Ph: +91-44-26680620, 26681266   Fax: +91-44-42032115   e-mail: chennai@cbspd.com
• **Kochi:** 42/1325, 1326, Power House Road, Opp. KSEB, Power House, Ernakulam 682018, Kochi, Kerala
  Ph: +91-484-4059061-65   Fax: +91-484-4059065   e-mail: kochi@cbspd.com
• **Kolkata:** 147, Hind Ceramics Compound, 1st Floor, Nilgunj Road, Belghoria, Kolkata-700056, West Bengal
  Ph: +91-9096713055/7798394118, 9836841399   e-mail: kolkata@cbspd.com
• **Lucknow:** Basement, Khushnuma Complex, 7-Meerabai Marg (Behind Jawahar Bhawan) Lucknow 226001, India
  Ph: 0522-4000032   e-mail: tiwari.lucknow@cbspd.com
• **Mumbai:** PWD Shed, Gala No. 25/26, Ramchandra Bhatt Marg, Next to JJ Hospital, Gate No. 2 Opp. Union Bank of India, Noorbaug, Mumbai 400009, Maharashtra, India
  Ph: +91-22-66661880/89   e-mail: mumbai@cbspd.com

Representatives

• **Hyderabad** 0-9885175004   • **Jharkhand** 0-9811541605   • **Nagpur**   0-9421945513
• **Patna**   0-9334159340   • **Pune**   0-9623451994   • **Uttarakhand** 0-9716462459

Printed at: Nutech Print Services, Faridabad, India

to

My beloved mother
Late Mrs Chintha Wijemanne

Foreword

Globally, 'single best answer (SBA)' questions are introduced with increasing frequency for undergraduate and postgraduate examinations. The students, as to be expected, find this relatively new method of assessment more difficult than the true/false multiple choice questions due to a dearth of books and model question papers to guide them.

Dr Samarakoon who is a senior teacher understood the difficulties faced by the students, when SBA questions were first introduced to the medical curriculum in Sri Lanka. She realized that successful preparation for an examination requires understanding the style and process of the examination. With these goals in mind she formulated a large number of questions and held many practice sessions to help the students to face the examination with confidence. This has helped the students of the Peradeniya University to achieve excellence at the final MBBS examination.

This book has a comprehensive collection of clinical principles, clinical scenario-based and knowledge-based questions, answers and explanations. It is a supplementary textbook covering the entire syllabus and not a mere collection of questions. The theory component of this book focuses directly on the clinical and practical knowledge required to answer SBA questions.

This book will be a great source of encouragement for medical students to face the final year examination with confidence, as they can practice answering diverse questions from every part of the syllabus. They can further facilitate their preparation, by using this book for revision and self-assessment prior to the examination.

This book is based on internationally accepted principles of patient management in accordance with the Guidelines of the Royal College of Obstetricians and Gynaecologists and the NICE Guidelines, with minimal adaptations to suit the clinical practice in Sri Lanka and other developing, low and middle income countries. Hence it is suitable for a large population of medical students in Sri Lanka and other Asian countries as well as for those in the UK and other Western countries.

Though the emphasis of the book is mainly on undergraduate education, it can also be used by postgraduate students preparing for the Doctor of Medicine in Obstetrics and Gynaecology (Sri Lanka), the MRCOG (UK) and other international examinations. It can be used even by lecturers as a guide to formulate new questions and to hold mock examinations and practice sessions.

There are very few books on standard SBA questions in gynaecology. This is the only book on SBA questions in gynaecology written by a Sri Lankan author. It is, in addition, a revision guide and almost a complete textbook suitable for a wide range of readers around the world and should be well accepted by undergraduate and even postgraduate students in Sri Lanka and abroad.

Prof **Vajira Weerasinghe** PhD (UK)
Dean, Faculty of Medicine,
University of Peradeniya,
Sri Lanka

Preface

This book is mainly intended as a supplementary textbook for medical students preparing for the final examination and for foreign medical graduates preparing for the Examination Required to Practice Medicine (ERPM) in Sri Lanka. However, it can be used for self-assessment and as a revision guide by postgraduate students, preparing for the doctor of medicine in obstetrics and gynaecology–part 2 (Sri Lanka), the MRCOG (UK) and other international postgraduate examinations. Since there are a large number of diverse questions, lecturers can use it as a guide to formulate new questions for examination papers and as an aid to conduct mock examinations and practise sessions.

The book contains 214 single best answer (SBA) questions, formulated from almost every possible clinical scenario in gynaecology. All the questions were formulated by me for the purpose of examination practice. A very detailed explanation is given for the correct answer, while the other four responses are critically discussed. The book is methodically arranged into 17 chapters. Each chapter contains a summary of the theory, questions, answers and explanations. The entire syllabus has been covered with questions from every part. The theory is focussed directly on the knowledge required to answer SBA questions.

The questions in this book are standard SBA questions, where all five responses are correct or at least plausible, but one response stands out among the rest as the correct answer. SBA questions are formulated mainly from basic clinical principles. These principles are included in the theory section and the more important ones are highlighted.

The theory is presented in an orderly sequence. It is essential for the student to study in an orderly manner as, "the next step in the management" and "the first line treatment" are commonly asked questions. Attention has been focused on the different types of questions asked at the end of the stem, as the average student will find it difficult to differentiate between these.

The book focuses on problem–based medicine and basic clinical principles, which form the basis of SBA questions. It is not merely a collection of SBA questions. To enable easy comprehension the theory is either in the form of a short summary or in the form of explanations for the answers. The explanations have been presented with the intent to enable the student to think logically and rationally to select the correct answer.

The main aim of compiling this book is to help the undergraduate and postgraduate students to face their examinations with confidence, as they can practice answering diverse questions from every part of the syllabus. My intent is to provide a complete guide for study purposes, examination practice and self-assessment. It can be used as a rapid revision guide as it summarises the entire syllabus in a compact manner.

It will be of great benefit for those sitting for the ERPM, as most students have not had an intensive clinical training and hence find it difficult to answer SBA questions, which are based on clinical scenarios.

Even though this book is intended as an aid for the written examination, it could be used by undergraduates and postgraduates as a guide for the OSCE and the practical clinical examination, because the questions describe a large number of clinical scenarios with the answers giving the appropriate management.

To my knowledge there is no book in the international market with a large collection of standard SBA questions in gynaecology, with detailed explanations for the answers, which focuses on the relevant theory as well. I have followed the Guidelines of the Royal College of Obstetricians and Gynaecologists and the National Institute for Health and Care Excellence (NICE), Guidelines (UK), with minimal deviations to suit the practise in Asian countries. Therefore, it is suitable for students in many countries around the world.

Two or three internationally accepted additional reading materials, which are relevant for both undergraduate and postgraduate students are given at the end of each chapter. I have given only a few very relevant references to minimise the time spent by students to obtain required information. The students are advised to read these to gather important information from which SBA questions can be formulated.

I am sure that this book will be helpful for undergraduates and postgraduates to face their examinations with confidence.

Eranthi Samarakoon

Acknowledgements

I am thankful to Prof Vajira Weerasinghe, Dean, Faculty of Medicine, University of Peradeniya, for encouraging me and writing the Foreword to this book.

I would like to acknowledge the guidance I received from the academic staff members of the Department of Obstetrics and Gynaecology, Faculty of Medicine, University of Peradeniya. A special word of thanks to Dr Chatura Rathnayaka and Dr Chandana Jayasundara for helping me with the final proofreading.

I very much appreciate the assistance of Mr Kamal Hemantha, the computer applications assistant of our department, who prepared the cover page and did the formatting and typesetting. He worked tirelessly to make this endeavour a success.

Finally I wish to thank all the academic staff members of the faculty, who helped me in numerous ways.

Eranthi Samarakoon

Contents

Abbreviations

ABST	Antibiotic sensitivity test		ICU	Intensive care unit
ACTH	Adrenocorticotropic hormone		IM	Intramuscular
AFP	Alpha fetoprotein		IOTA study	International Ovarian Tumour Analysis (IOTA) group
AGC	Abnormal glandular cells		IU	International units
AIS	Adenocarcinoma *in situ*		IUCD	Intrauterine contraceptive device
AUB	Abnormal uterine bleeding		LDH	Lactate dehydrogenase
BMI	Body mass index		LH	Luteinising hormone
bpm	Beats per minute		LNGIUS	Levonorgestrel-releasing intra-uterine system
cm	Centimetres			
CNS	Central nervous system		LSIL	Low-grade squamous intraepithelial lesion
CRL	Crown-rump length			
DES	Diethylstilbestrol		mcg	Micrograms
DIC	Disseminated intravascular coagulation		mg	Milligrams
			mm	Millimetres
DMPA	Depot medroxyprogesterone acetate		NSAIDs	Nonsteroidal anti-inflammatory drugs
ELISA	Enzyme linkedimmunosorbent assay		OCP	Oral contraceptive pills
			OGTT	Oral glucose tolerance test
FIGO	International Federation of Gynaecology and Obstetrics		PCOS	Polycystic ovarian syndrome
			PCR	Polymerase chain reaction
FSH	Follicular stimulating hormone		PID	Pelvic inflammatory disease
GnRH	Gonadotropin releasing hormone		POA	Period of amenorrhoea
			RCOG	Royal College of Obstetricians & Gynaecologists
GTD	Gestational trophoblastic disease			
GTN	Gestational trophoblastic neoplasia		RMI	Risk of malignancy index
			SCJ	Squamocolumnar junction
hCG	Human chorionic gonadotropin		SLCOG	Sri Lanka College of Obstetricians and Gynaecologists
HIV	Human immunodeficiency virus			
HMB	Heavy menstrual bleeding			
HPV	Human papillomavirus		STI	Sexually transmitted infections
HRT	Hormone replacement therapy		TSH	Thyroid stimulating hormone
HSIL	High grade squamous intraepithelial lesion		TVUS/TVS	Transvaginal ultrasound scan
			USS	Ultrasound scan
ICSI	Intracytoplasmic sperm injection		VDRL test	Venereal disease research laboratory (VDRL) test

Guidelines for Answering Single Best Answer Type Questions

Single best answer (SBA) questions are based on the management of "real" patients who have common clinical conditions. *Therefore, a sound clinical and practical knowledge is necessary to score high marks.*

These questions are not based on *recall* of knowledge, but on *application* of knowledge.

Single best answer (SBA) questions are based on the basic clinical principles. These principles are given in the short summaries of each chapter. The most important areas are highlighted.

The stem of each question will give a summary of a common clinical condition, with a definite diagnosis, which will be obvious. There will be no uncertainty or ambiguity. Therefore, the student should not try to read "in between the lines".

The information given in the stem is adequate to answer the question.

The student should take into consideration only the information given in the question. He should not add more data from his knowledge. He must consider only the patient information given in the stem. He should not think about a similar patient he has managed in the ward, as there may be many important differences between the two. His mind should be clear and he should focus his attention only on the information given in the stem.

A question will be asked at the end of the stem and five responses will be given. The responses are arranged in the alphabetical order.

In a good SBA question all five responses will be plausible and even correct, but one response will stand out as the *correct* answer.

In a good SBA question the "cover test should be positive". If the question is read after covering the responses, the correct answer should be obvious.

The common questions which are asked at the end of the stem are:

- What is the most appropriate management?
- What is the next step/first step in the management?
- What is the first line treatment?

What is the most appropriate management?

The answer expected for this question is the standard clinical management.

Examples

- Performing a hysterectomy for a 40-year-old multiparous woman with a large fibroid uterus.
- Performing a cruciate incision in the hymen for the treatment of cryptomenorrhoea due to an imperforate hymen.
- Performing laparoscopic ovarian cystectomy for a benign ovarian cyst in a woman of reproductive age.
- Performing suction evacuation for a hydatidiform mole.
- Treating chlamydial infection with doxycycline.
- Performing a loop electrosurgical excision to treat CIN 2.

What is the first step in the management/ the first line treatment?

The immediate management of the patient will be the correct answer to this question. This would include carrying out a crucial investigation or the initial treatment.

Examples

- Performing a transvaginal ultrasound scan in a woman with postmenopausal bleeding.
- Carrying out expectant management for a missed abortion.

- Treating a woman with regular heavy menstrual bleeding without structural abnormalities with tranexamic acid.
- Medical treatment for parous patients with endometriosis.

What is the next step in the management?

The question should be carefully read as the next step begins at the end of the question. It could be an investigation or the next step in the treatment.

Examples

- Performing serum beta hCG levels in a woman with a positive urine hCG test and no IUP on the transvaginal scan.
- Performing serial beta hCG levels weekly after evacuating a hydatidiform mole.
- Giving radiotherapy after surgery for stage IB endometrial carcinoma.

To answer this type of questions the student should have a clear knowledge of the sequence of events in managing common clinical conditions.

The knowledge required to answer SBA questions should be acquired by managing patients during the clinical appointment. Notes and information obtained from ward teaching sessions and lectures are also important as these emphasize mainly on patient management.

Reading material should include mainly the clinical guidelines of the Royal College of Obstetricians and Gynaecologists, the NICE (National Institute for Health and Care Excellence, UK) Guidelines and the local guidelines of your country. A standard textbook recommended by your medical faculty may be used.

Extra reading will not be very useful and can cause confusion, as there could be subtle differences regarding patient management in different countries and in different books.

Two or three relevant references which should be read by the students are given at the end of each chapter. The students are advised to read these references to gather important information from which SBA questions can be formulated.

1

Abnormal Uterine Bleeding

NORMAL MENSTRUAL PERIOD

The average interval between menstrual cycles is 28 days, but it can range from 21 to 35 days. The normal duration of bleeding is 3 to 5 days. The amount should be less than 80 ml (less than 1 pad or tampon per 3-hour period).

Abnormal uterine bleeding (AUB) includes menstrual bleeding that is abnormally heavy or occurs outside the normal cyclic menstruation (abnormal in timing).

- The term dysfunctional uterine bleeding was earlier used for bleeding caused by non-structural entities such as coagulopathy, endometrial dysfunction, and ovulatory disorders (Fig. 1.1).

- **Heavy menstrual bleeding (HMB)** should replace menorrhagia to describe excessive cyclical menstrual bleeding of more than 80 ml per period. Bleeding can be excessive for the normal duration (soaking a pad or tampon more than once in two hours) or last longer than 5 days.

- **Intermenstrual bleeding** occurs between clearly defined cyclic menstruations and should replace the term metorrhagia.

- **Irregular bleeding** is menstruation which occurs at intervals of less than 21 days and more than 35 days. This includes inter-menstrual bleeding, oligomenorrhoea, prolonged bleeding that can last weeks or months, and other irregular patterns.

- If the bleeding is consistently **postcoital**, this suggests cervical pathology, including cervical neoplasia. However, postcoital bleeding may occur with contact during intercourse of any site along the lower genital tract that is friable (e.g. due to cervicitis or vulvovaginal atrophy) or has a lesion (e.g. cervical polyp or vulvar ulcer.)

- **Frequent menstrual bleeding** is occurrence of more than 4 episodes of bleeding during a period of 90 days.

- **Infrequent menstruation** is occurrence of 1–2 episodes of bleeding in 90 days.

- **Amenorrhoea** is the absence of menstruation for 90 days. (This is different from secondary amenorrhoea which is a pathological entity.)

- **Chronic AUB** is defined as bleeding from the uterine corpus that is abnormal in volume, regularity, or timing and has been present for most of the prior 6 months.

- **Acute AUB** is defined as an episode of heavy bleeding requiring immediate intervention.

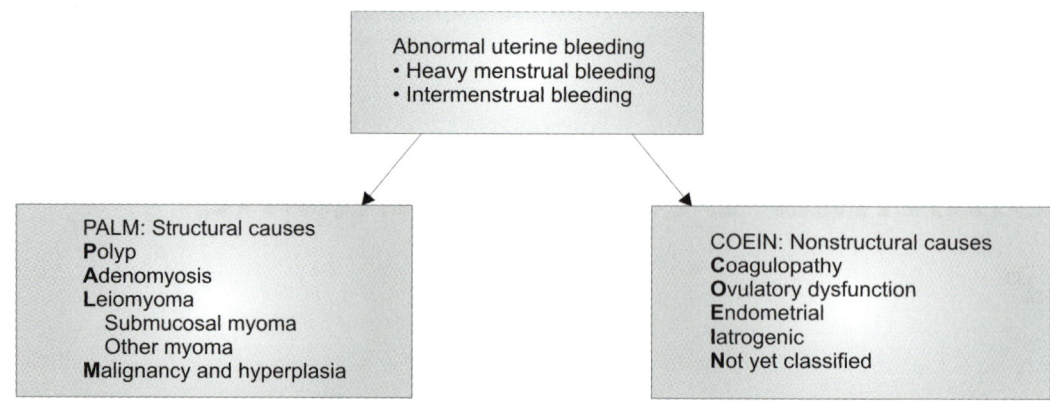

Fig. 1.1: Causes of abnormal uterine bleeding

The classification system does not include abnormal bleeding related to pathological conditions of the lower reproductive tract.

- Age is an important factor because the aetiology differs in different age groups.
- In the adolescent age group (under 20 years) structural defects are unlikely to be present and non-structural causes in the COEIN group should be considered. The commonest causative factor is ovulatory dysfunction.
- In the perimenopausal age group (over 40 years) any of the above causes can occur, but ovulatory dysfunction is common and malignancy should be excluded.
- Heavy menstrual bleeding is caused by fibroids, adenomyosis, bleeding disorders, endometrial polyps, endometrial hyperplasia, arteriovenous malformations in the uterus, local disorders of haemostasis in the uterus and copper containing intrauterine devices.
- Irregular menstrual bleeding is caused by endometrial polyps, endometrial hyperplasia, malignancy, pelvic inflammatory disease, ovulatory dysfunction (usually with longer intervals), use of gonadal steroids and cervical and lower genital tract lesions. The latter 2 also cause postcoital bleeding.

THE PALM GROUP

Polyps
- Include endometrial or endocervical polyps.
- May be symptomless or may cause heavy menstrual bleeding (endometrial polyps), irregular bleeding, postcoital bleeding or vaginal discharge.
- Diagnosed by transvaginal ultrasound scanning and will be seen as an area of focal thickening of the endometrium.
- Diagnosis is confirmed by hysteroscopy and resection can be carried out at the same time.

Adenomyosis
- Causes heavy menstrual bleeding with dysmenorrhoea and dyspareunia.
- Diagnosed by bimanual examination and transvaginal ultrasound scanning.
- On examination the uterus is tender and uniformly enlarged.
- Ultrasound scanning will show uniform hypertrophy of the myometrium with diffuse myometrial lesions.

Leiomyoma
- Generally mainly submucosal tumours cause heavy menstrual loss. Intramural fibroids also can cause HMB due to distortion and altered contractility of the myometrium. It

can also cause increased vascularity of the myometrium extending to the submucosal layer.

Malignancy or Endometrial Hyperplasia

- These conditions cause irregular bleeding. Endometrial hyperplasia can cause HMB.

THE COIN GROUP

Coagulopathy

- Can be due to blood disorders such as von Willebrand disease or anti-coagulant treatment.
- Causes HMB or irregular bleeding.

Ovulatory Dysfunction

- Can cause amenorrhoea, scanty bleeding, unpredictable and irregular bleeding or heavy menstrual bleeding.
- The cause of dysfunction may be ill-defined or may be due to PCOS, hyperprolacti-naemia, hypothyroidism, mental stress, obesity, weight loss, anorexia or excessive exercise.
- More common at extremes of reproductive age such as adolescence and the perimeno-pausal period.

Endometrial Disorder

- A diagnosis is reached after excluding other causes.
- The disorder may occur due to local production of vasodilators, reduced production of vasoconstrictors and increased production of lytic substances.

Iatrogenic Causes

- Amenorrhoea, breakthrough bleeding and irregular bleeding can be caused by combined oral contraceptives, injectable progestogen preparations, progestogen implants and levonorgestrel containing intrauterine devices. Copper containing intrauterine devices can cause excessive and/or irregular bleeding.

- Phenothiazine, tricyclic anti-depressants, anti-psychotic drugs such as risperidone, can cause reduced inhibition of prolactin release, resulting in amenorrhoea and irregular bleeding.
- Phenytoin, corticosteroids and tamoxifen also can cause abnormal uterine bleeding.

INVESTIGATION OF A PATIENT WITH ABNORMAL UTERINE BLEEDING

- Exclude pregnancy.
- Exclude post-menopausal bleeding.
- Confirm the chronic nature.
- Exclude structural causes.
- Consider non-structural causes.

History

- Age is an important factor because the aetiology differs in different age groups.
- Exclude pregnancy by history of a period of amenorrhoea, symptoms of pregnancy and a positive urine or serum beta hCG test.
- Consider postmenopausal bleeding, if there is a period of amenorrhoea of more than 1 year in a woman older than 45 years.
- Exclude iatrogenic causes.
- Assess the amount of bleeding. Heavy menstruation is considered as soaking a pad or tampon more than every two hours or as a volume of bleeding that interferes with daily activities (e.g. wakes patient from sleep, stains clothing or sheets).
- Consider the pattern of bleeding. Leiomyoma and adenomyosis will cause excessive menstrual bleeding while adenomyosis will cause dysmenorrhoea as well. Endocervical and endometrial polyps and endometrial carcinoma will cause irregular bleeding with intermittent discharge though endometrial polyps can also cause HMB. Ovulatory dysfunction will cause irregular bleeding after a prolonged interval. Irregular use of hormonal contraceptives will cause totally irregular and unpredictable bleeding.

- Postcoital bleeding is caused by cervical and lower genital tract lesions.
- Consider accompanying symptoms such as dysmenorrhoea which may be present in endometriosis, adenomyosis and pelvic inflammatory disease.
- Exclude symptoms suggestive of systemic causes of bleeding such as hypothyroidism, hyperprolactinaemia, coagulation disorders, liver disease, adrenal or hypothalamic disorders.
- Exclude symptoms of PCOS such as obesity, hirsutism and infertility.
- Exclude a family history or personal history of a coagulation disorder.
- Symptoms of anaemia may be present.
- History of previous investigations and previous treatment should be taken.

Examination

- General examination for:
    - pallor of the mucous membrane in anaemia,
    - petechiae and lymphadenopathy in coagulation disorders,
    - obesity and hirsutism in PCOS.
- Abdominal examination for:
    - masses in leiomyoma and adenomyosis.
- Speculum examination to identify:
    - lower genital tract lesions,
    - endocervical polyps,
    - threads of an IUCD.
- Bimanual examination to determine the size of the uterus.
    - The uterus will be enlarged in leiomyoma, adenomyosis and disturbed pregnancy states.
    - The enlargement may be smooth or irregular in leiomyoma while the enlargement is smooth and less than 16 weeks in size in adenomyosis.
    - Uterine enlargement will be absent or minimal in endometrial carcinoma.

Investigations

- Full blood count.
- Coagulation profile if a coagulation disorder is suspected.
- Pituitary gonadotropin levels and prolactin levels are done in patients with oligomenorrhoea and suspected anovulation.
- Thyroid function tests are done only if a disorder is suspected.
- Transvaginal ultrasound scanning:
    - is done to diagnose fibroids, adenomyosis, endometrial polyps, endometrial hyperplasia and endometrial carcinoma.
    - is a very useful investigation and should be done in all cases, if a structural lesion is suspected.
    - should always be done in all women over the age of 35 years and in cases not responding to medical management.
- The normal endometrium in a premenopausal woman varies in thickness according to the menstrual cycle, from 4 mm in the follicular phase, up to 16 mm in the luteal phase.
    - during menstruation 2–4 mm
    - early proliferative phase (days 6–14): 5–7 mm
    - late proliferative-preovulatory phase: Up to 11 mm
    - secretory phase: 7–16 mm
- In premenopausal women, measurement of endometrial thickness is not a useful test, since major variations of the thickness occur during the normal menstrual cycle. However, transvaginal ultrasound can identify structural causes of AUB and focal thickening of the endometrium due to hyperplasia or cancer.
- Endometrial thickness should be less than 5 mm in a post-menopausal woman.
- Saline infusion sonohysterogram:
    - is done if uterine pathology is suspected, especially to confirm submucous fibroids or endometrial polyps.

- Endometrial biopsy should be done in women over the age of 45 years if:
  - increased endometrial thickness is diagnosed on transvaginal ultrasound scanning,
  - there is significant and persistent inter-menstrual, irregular or heavy menstrual bleeding,
  - the bleeding is not responding to medical management.
- Endometrial biopsy is considered in women under the age of 45 years if:
  - there are risk factors for endometrial carcinoma,
  - there is unopposed exposure to oestrogens with increased endometrial thickness as in PCOS,
  - the bleeding is not responding to medical management.
- Office endometrial biopsy is performed as an outpatient procedure.
- Hysteroscopy and biopsy is recommended if irregular endometrial thickening or a focal lesion is diagnosed on transvaginal scanning and in cases of postmenopausal bleeding.

TREATMENT

- If a structural lesion is found appropriate, treatment should be carried out (will be discussed in the relevant chapters).
- If the bleeding is due to irregular use of hormonal contraceptives, regular use should be recommended or the method should be changed.
- Anaemia should be treated.
- Medical treatment is the first line treatment for those without a structural lesion.
- Medical treatment is selected according to the woman's age, desire for contraception, underlying medical conditions and contraindications and tolerance of side effects.
- Those with coagulation disorders will need concomitant factor replacement.

MEDICAL TREATMENT FOR ABNORMAL UTERINE BLEEDING

- **Non-hormonal**
  - Non-steroidal anti-inflammatory drugs
  - Antifibrinolytic drugs
- **Hormonal**
  - Combined oral contraceptive pills
  - Levonorgestrel-releasing intrauterine system
  - Oral norethisterone
  - Oral medroxyprogesterone acetate
  - Danazol
  - GnRH-agonists

Non-hormonal Treatment

Regular, heavy menstrual bleeding can be treated with non-hormonal methods.

- **Non-steroidal anti-inflammatory drugs (NSAIDs) and antifibrinolytics**
  - These can be used alone or in combination to treat regular heavy menstrual bleeding.
  - They will reduce the amount or duration of bleeding but will not stop irregular bleeding.
  - Treatment should be commenced on the first day of bleeding and continued for the duration of the flow.
  - NSAIDs reduce total prostaglandin production through the inhibition of cyclo-oxygenase, shifting the balance between prostaglandins and thromboxanes to promote uterine vasoconstriction.
  - Mefenamic acid and naproxen are commonly used but other NSAIDs are also effective.
  - NSAIDs relieve dysmenorrhoea as well.
  - Women with heavy menstrual bleeding have been found to have elevated endometrial levels of plasminogen activators, with more local fibrinolytic activity.
  - Tranexamic acid is an antifibrinolytic agent (or plasminogen activator inhibitor) which reduces the menstrual

blood loss. It can be used alone or in combination with NSAIDs. It has no effect on dysmenorrhoea. Intravenous preparation can be used if there is acute blood loss.

Hormonal Treatment

- Is recommended for those with irregular bleeding in the absence of a structural lesion and for those with heavy menstrual bleeding without a structural lesion, who are not responding to treatment with non-hormonal methods.
- Combined oral contraceptive pills, oral norethisterone, oral medroxyprogesterone acetate, and levonorgestrel-releasing intra-uterine systems, significantly reduce menstrual bleeding and should be used to treat women with abnormal uterine bleeding.
- Combined oral contraceptive pills are administered cyclically in the same manner as for contraception, though resistant cases may need double the normal dose.
- Norethisterone is administered cyclically, in a dose of 5 mg twice or thrice daily for 21 days, followed by a treatment free period of 7 days, before commencing the next cycle.
- Oral medroxyprogesterone acetate 10 mg 3 times daily for 14 days, from the 14th day of the cycle, with 14 days off treatment is also an option.
- The minimum duration of treatment for the above methods is at least one cycle, but usually treatment is continued for 3 cycles.
- Combined oral contraceptive pills and norethisterone are equally effective, but combined oral contraceptive pills are preferred because they are cheap and freely available. Also they are available in a calendar pack and have the convenience of once daily administration. Norethisterone is the preferred option for women over the age of 40 years and for those who have contraindications for OCP.

- Depot medroxyprogesterone acetate injections are usually not used because of the high incidence of prolonged amenorrhoea and breakthrough bleeding.
- Levonorgestrel-releasing intrauterine system is the ideal method for women over the age of 40 years, who need effective contraception as well. It can be used as an alternative for hysterectomy. Sometimes it can cause breakthrough bleeding.
- Danazol and gonadotropin-releasing hormone agonists will effectively reduce menstrual bleeding, but are not usually used due to side effects.

SURGICAL TREATMENT

The indications for surgery
- Presence of uterine pathology.
- Presence of atypical endometrial hyper-plasia/risk of endometrial carcinoma.
- Failure to respond to medical therapy/contraindications for medical treatment.
- Significant anaemia needing blood transfusion.

Surgical options include:
- hysteroscopic polypectomy,
- endometrial ablation,
- myomectomy,
- hysterectomy.
- Hysteroscopic polypectomy is carried out for endometrial and endocervical polyps.
- Endometrial ablation is a minimally invasive surgical option for heavy menstrual bleeding. It may be considered in women who have not responded to medical treatment, have completed childbearing, not at risk of endometrial carcinoma and do not have structural lesions requiring major surgery.
- Myomectomy is carried out for large or symptomatic fibroids in women who wish to preserve their fertility.

UTERINE FIBROIDS

Uterine fibroids may be symptomless or may cause:

- heavy menstrual bleeding, more frequently with submucous tumours,
- an abdominal/pelvic mass,
- pressure symptoms on the renal system or the bowel,
- infertility.
- Pain is not common but may occur in fibroid polyps, torsion of the pedicle of a subserous pedunculated fibroid, degeneration or sarcomatous change.

Fibroids cause a firm, smooth or irregular uterine enlargement which could reach a large size.

The diagnosis is confirmed by ultrasound scanning. Discreet tumours can be seen.

Complications

- Torsion of a pedunculated subserous fibroid.
- Infection of a submucous myoma.
- Malignant change in 0.2% of uterine fibroids.
- Degeneration (hyaline/cystic/fatty/red degeneration). Red degeneration occurs only during pregnancy. It causes pain which could even be severe, vomiting and mild fever. It is treated symptomatically.

TREATMENT

Small symptomless fibroids do not require treatment. Asymptomatic fibroids may warrant treatment in the following situations:

- The size of the fibroid uterus is more than a 12–14 weeks pregnant uterus.
- Rapid growth of the tumour.
- Evidence of hydroureter/hydronephrosis caused by compression of ureters by the tumour.
- Subserous pedunculated fibroids are liable to undergo torsion of the pedicle and hence may be treated even if asymptomatic.

Medical Management

- Heavy menstrual bleeding caused by small submucous fibroids can be treated with mefenamic acid, combined oral contraceptive pills, oral progestogens or LNG/IUS (if the uterine cavity is not distorted).
- GnRH analogues are used to reduce the size and vascularity of fibroids prior to surgery.

Uterine Artery Embolization

- Can be offered for symptomatic fibroids.
- Is contraindicated in the presence of pelvic infection, pregnancy, or if there is a doubt regarding the possibility of malignancy.
- The patient should accept the small risk of needing a hysterectomy if complications occur.
- It has the advantage of shorter hospital stay and quicker return to normal activities.
- The fertility rates are almost similar to that following myomectomy.

Hysteroscopic Resection/Morcellation

- Is recommended for submucous fibroids less than 5 cm in diameter.
- The procedure is carried out under general or spinal anaesthesia.
- Complications include fluid overload, infection, uterine perforation, bowel damage and spread of an undiagnosed malignancy. Hysteroscopic morcellators do not pose the same risk as laparoscopic power morcellators, because any sarcomatous tissue present will not enter the peritoneal cavity.

Myomectomy

- Myomectomy by laparoscopy or laparotomy is indicated in those with symptomatic or large fibroids, who have fertility wishes.
- Profuse bleeding can occur during the procedure as fibroids are enucleated from the capsule. Haemostasis is achieved by diathermy cauterisation and application of deep mattress sutures.

- At least 3 pints of blood should be cross-matched and consent should be taken for hysterectomy.
- It is necessary to open into the endometrial cavity if submucous fibroids are present. If this is done there is a high risk of uterine rupture during a subsequent delivery.

Therefore, a caesarean section has to be performed.

Hysterectomy

Hysterectomy is the treatment for large or symptomatic fibroids in women who do not have fertility wishes.

QUESTIONS

1. **A 46-year-old woman complains of continuous vaginal bleeding for two months. No abnormalities are detected on abdominal and vaginal examination.**

   What is the next step in the management?

   A. Insertion of a levonorgestrel-releasing intrauterine device.

   B. Hysteroscopy and biopsy.

   C. Pipelle aspiration.

   D. Therapeutic trial with norethisterone.

   E. Transvaginal ultrasound scanning.

2. **A 40-year-old multiparous woman complains of frequent irregular vaginal bleeding for two months. Abdominal and vaginal examinations are normal. Transvaginal ultrasound scan reveals an endometrial thickness of 8 mm with no other abnormalities. The haemoglobin percentage is 10 g/dl and the platelet count is within the normal range.**

   What is the best treatment option?

   A. Administer combined oral contraceptive pills for 3 cycles.

   B. Administer norethisterone 5 mg three times daily for 3 cycles.

   C. Insert a levonorgestrel-releasing intrauterine device.

   D. Perform endometrial ablation.

   E. Perform an endometrial biopsy.

3. **A 42-year-old multiparous woman complains of irregular bleeding for two months. Abdominal and vaginal examinations are normal. Transvaginal ultrasound scan reveals an endometrial thickness of 17 mm. Endometrial biopsy reveals simple endometrial hyperplasia without atypia. The haemoglobin percentage is 9 g/dl.**

   What is the best treatment option?

   A. Administer combined oral contraceptive pills for 3 cycles.

   B. Administer norethisterone 5 mg three times daily for 3 cycles.

   C. Insert a levonorgestrel-releasing intrauterine device.

   D. Perform endometrial ablation.

   E. Perform a hysterectomy.

4. **A 50-year-old nulliparous woman with diabetes mellitus complains of heavy irregular bleeding for six months. Abdominal and vaginal examinations are normal. Transvaginal ultrasound scan reveals an endometrial thickness of 8 mm with no other abnormalities. The haemoglobin percentage is 9 g/dl. Her BMI is 30.**

   What is the next step in the management?

   A. Hysteroscopic visualisation and biopsy.

   B. Insert a levonorgestrel-releasing intrauterine device.

   C. Perform pipelle aspiration.

   D. Perform a hysterectomy.

   E. Perform endometrial ablation.

5. **A 17-year-old girl complains of continuous vaginal bleeding for 3 weeks.**

She has had two previous similar episodes. Her BMI is 20. She has mild pallor of the mucus membranes, but no other abnormalities are detected. The haemoglobin percentage is 9 g/dl. The coagulation profile and the ultrasound scan are normal.

What is the most appropriate treatment?

A. Cyclical treatment with oral contraceptive pills for 3 months.

B. Norethisterone 5 mg thrice daily for 10 days.

C. Norethisterone 5 mg twice daily for 3 cycles of 21 days.

D. Oral iron therapy.

E. Tranexamic acid 500 mg 8 hourly for 1 week.

6. A 17-year-old girl complains of heavy menstrual bleeding for 6 months. She has severe dysmenorrhoea on the first day of menstruation. She has 28-day regular cycles with excessive flow for 5 days. No abnormalities are detected on examination. The haemoglobin percentage is 9 g/dl. The coagulation profile and the ultrasound scan are normal.

What is the most appropriate first line treatment?

A. Oral contraceptive pills for 3 cycles.

B. Mefenamic acid 500 mg 8 hourly during menstruation.

C. Norethisterone 5 mg three times daily for 7 days during menstruation.

D. Norethisterone 5 mg twice daily for 3 cycles of 21 days.

E. Tranexamic acid 500 mg 8 hourly during menstruation.

7. A 35-year-old woman complains of heavy menstrual bleeding for 6 months. She has 28-day regular cycles which last for 7 days. Abdominal and vaginal examinations are normal. The haemoglobin percentage is 9 g/dl and the platelet count is within the normal range. The transvaginal ultrasound scan is normal.

What is the most appropriate first line treatment?

A. Cyclical treatment with oral contraceptive pills for 3 months.

B. Dilatation and curettage.

C. Norethisterone 5 mg three times daily for 7 days during menstruation.

D. Norethisterone 5 mg twice daily for 3 cycles of 21 days.

E. Tranexamic acid 500 mg 8 hourly for 1 week during menstruation.

7a. A 36-year-old woman complains of irregular frequent menstrual bleeding for 6 months. Abdominal and vaginal examinations are normal. The haemoglobin level is 9 g/dl and the platelet count is normal. The transvaginal ultrasound scan is normal. Her BMI is 30.

What is the most appropriate first line treatment?

A. Cyclical treatment with oral contraceptive pills for 3 months.

B. Dilatation and curettage.

C. Norethisterone 5 mg three times daily for 7 days during menstruation.

D. Norethisterone 5 mg twice daily for 3 cycles of 21 days.

E. Tranexamic acid 500 mg 8 hourly for 1 week during menstruation.

8. A 48-year-old woman complains of irregular, frequent heavy menstrual bleeding for 2 months. Abdominal and vaginal examinations are normal. Transvaginal ultrasound scan reveals an endometrial polyp.

What is the most appropriate treatment?

A. Dilatation and curettage.

B. Endometrial ablation.

C. Hysterectomy.

D. Hysteroscopic resection of the polyp.

E. Polypectomy by hysterotomy.

9. A 44-year-old woman complains of continuous vaginal bleeding for 6 months. She has had an endometrial biopsy 3 months ago and the histology report revealed proliferative endometrium. She responded to treatment with norethisterone 5 mg twice daily for 3 cycles of 21 days, but bleeding recurred soon after cessation of treatment. Transvaginal ultrasound scan reveals an endometrial thickness of 8 mm. The haemoglobin level is 9.5 gm/dl. The platelet count is normal. Her BMI is 22. She does not have any medical complications.

    What is the most appropriate method of treatment?

    A. Insert a levonorgestrel-releasing intrauterine system.
    B. Perform a hysterectomy.
    C. Perform a dilatation and curettage.
    D. Perform endometrial ablation.
    E. Treat with oral contraceptive pills for 3 cycles.

9a. A 44-year-old woman complains of continuous vaginal bleeding for 6 months. She has had an endometrial biopsy 3 months ago and the histology report revealed proliferative endometrium. She did not respond to medical treatment with norethisterone 5 mg twice daily 21 days. Transvaginal ultrasound scan reveals an endometrial thickness of 9 mm. The haemoglobin level is 9 gm/dl. The platelet count is normal.

    What is the most appropriate method of treatment?

    A. Insert a levonorgestrel-releasing intrauterine system.
    B. Perform a dilatation and curettage.
    C. Perform a hysterectomy.
    D. Perform endometrial ablation.
    E. Treat with oral contraceptive pills for 3 cycles.

10. A 35-year-old woman complains of heavy menstrual bleeding for 1 year. She has one child, 6 years of age. Her haemoglobin level is 8.5 g/dl. Ultrasound scan reveals a single 3 cm × 3 cm submucosal fibroid.

    What is the best treatment option?

    A. Administer oral norethisterone continuously for 3 months.
    B. Perform hysteroscopic morcellation.
    C. Perform uterine artery embolization.
    D. Perform hysteroscopic resection.
    E. Perform laparoscopic myomectomy.

11. A 43-year-old woman presents with heavy menstrual bleeding. She has one child 6 years of age. The uterus is enlarged to 24 weeks with multiple fibroids. Her haemoglobin level is 9 g/dl.

    What is the best treatment option?

    A. Monthly injection of GnRH analogues for 3 months followed by myomectomy.
    B. Myomectomy followed by monthly injection of GnRH analogues for 3 months.
    C. Hysterectomy and bilateral salpingo-oophorectomy followed by HRT.
    D. Hysterectomy with preservation of both ovaries.
    E. Uterine artery embolization.

12. A 43-year-old nulliparous woman presents with heavy irregular menstrual bleeding. Abdominal examination is normal. Speculum examination reveals a large fibroid polyp protruding through the cervical os. No other fibroids are detected on the ultrasound scan.

    What is the best treatment option?

    A. Abdominal hysterectomy.
    B. Hysteroscopic resection.
    C. Myomectomy by laparotomy.
    D. Uterine artery embolization.
    E. Vaginal myomectomy (polypectomy).

13. A 43-year-old multiparous woman presents with heavy menstrual bleeding and dysmenorrhoea which outlast the period. Abdominal and vaginal examinations reveal a uniformly enlarged uterus, corresponding in size to 14 weeks. Ultrasound examination reveals a uniformly enlarged uterus with marked myometrial thickening.

    What is the most appropriate treatment?

    A. Perform a hysterectomy.

    B. Treat with Danazol for 6 months.

    C. Treat with depot medroxyprogesterone acetate injections once a month for 6 months.

    D. Treat with GnRH analogues for 3 months.

    E. Treat with Mefenamic and Tranexamic acid during the menstrual period.

14. A 46-year-old woman complains of irregular bleeding for two months. No abnormalities are detected on abdominal and vaginal examination. Transvaginal ultrasound scan reveals an endometrial thickness of 15 mm. Endometrial biopsy reveals atypical endometrial hyperplasia.

    What is the best treatment option?

    A. Insert a levonorgestrel-releasing intra-uterine device.

    B. Perform a total hysterectomy and bilateral salpingectomy.

    C. Perform a total hysterectomy and bilateral salpingo-oophorectomy.

    D. Perform a total hysterectomy, bilateral salpingectomy and pelvic lymphadenectomy.

    E. Perform endometrial ablation.

15. A 45-year-old multiparous woman complains of irregular bleeding for two months. No abnormalities are detected on abdominal and vaginal examination. Transvaginal ultrasound scan reveals uniform thickening of the endometrium measuring 12 mm. What is the next step in the management?

    A. Dilatation and curettage

    B. Hysteroscopic visualisation and biopsy.

    C. MRI scan.

    D. Outpatient endometrial biopsy (pipelle aspiration).

    E. Saline infusion sonohysterography.

16. A 46-year-old woman complains of irregular bleeding for two months. No abnormalities are detected on abdominal and vaginal examination. Transvaginal ultrasound scan reveals irregular thickening of the endometrium with a maximum thickness of 14 mm.

    What is the next step in the management?

    A. Dilatation and curettage

    B. Hysteroscopic visualisation and biopsy.

    C. MRI scan.

    D. Outpatient endometrial biopsy.

    E. Saline infusion sonohysterography.

ANSWERS AND EXPLANATIONS

Q. 1 (E)

The possibility of a structural lesion or endometrial malignancy should be considered, because the woman is more than 45 years of age and has continuous bleeding. Therefore, the next step in the management is to perform a transvaginal ultrasound scan, to exclude structural lesions which can cause continuous bleeding, such as endometrial polyps, endometrial hyperplasia and endometrial carcinoma. Hysteroscopy or pipelle aspiration is performed to confirm the diagnosis of endometrial hyperplasia or endometrial carcinoma suspected by the ultrasound scan. Insertion of a LNGIUS or treatment with norethisterone is commenced only after excluding structural lesions.

Q. 2 (C)

Since no structural or other abnormalities have been found, the bleeding is most probably due to ovulatory dysfunction, which is common in women over the age of 40 years. Insertion of a levonorgestrel-releasing intrauterine device is the best option, as it will provide long-term treatment as well as effective contraception. Oral norethisterone can be used, but the woman has to take treatment regularly (or there will be breakthrough bleeding) and the treatment is short term. OCP is best avoided in women over the age of 35 years. Endometrial biopsy is not necessary as the endometrial thickness is normal on TVUS and there are no risk factors for endometrial carcinoma. It should be performed if medical treatment fails. Endometrial ablation is considered only if medical treatment fails.

Q. 3 (C)

The risk of endometrial hyperplasia without atypia progressing to endometrial cancer is less than 5% over 20 years and the majority will regress spontaneously during follow-up. Therefore, endometrial ablation or hysterectomy is not necessary. Observation alone with follow-up endo-metrial biopsies, to ensure disease regre-ssion is recommended in women without symptoms and who are at low risk of endometrial carcinoma. Treatment with progesterone is indicated in this woman as she has bleeding. Also progesterone will cause regression of the hyperplasia.

Insertion of a levonorgestrel-releasing intrauterine device is the best treatment option, because compared to oral proges-terone it is more effective to control bleeding and to cause regression of the hyperplasia. It will also provide effective contraception. It has fewer side effects. If oral norethisterone is given, the treatment should be given continuously for 6 months. Cyclical treatment should not be used because it is less effective in inducing regression of endometrial hyperplasia.

Q. 4 (A)

This patient is at high risk of endometrial carcinoma due to the history of prolonged irregular bleeding, age, obesity, diabetes and nulliparity. Therefore, hysteroscopic visualisation of the endometrial cavity and biopsy is preferred to pipelle aspiration. It is the next step in the management and should be performed before commencing treatment, even though the transvaginal scan is normal. If the histology does not reveal hyperplasia or malignancy, medical management with a levonorgestrel-releasing intrauterine device is the best option. Treatment with oral norethisterone is another option. Hysterectomy also should be considered because she has several risk factors for endometrial carcinoma. Endometrial ablation should be avoided because complete and persistent endometrial destruction cannot be ensured and intrauterine adhesion formation may preclude endometrial histological surveillance.

Q. 5 (A)

Structural abnormalities are unlikely because she is an adolescent girl and the USS is normal. The coagulation profile is normal and she is not on any drugs. Therefore, bleeding is due to ovulatory dysfunction and she should be treated with hormones. OCP or oral progesterone can be used. OCP is the preferred option because it is cheap, freely available, comes in a calendar pack and is usually administered once daily. Whatever hormone is used treatment should be continued for at least 3 cycles, to obtain satisfactory control. Treatment with progestogen during the luteal phase is less effective in maintaining cyclical control. Tranexamic acid is used to reduce heavy menstrual bleeding, but will not stop continuous or irregular bleeding. Oral iron should be given to restore the haemoglobin level.

Q. 6 (B)

Since she has heavy menstrual bleeding and dysmenorrhoea, the best option is treatment with mefenamic acid. Treatment is commenced on the first day of menstruation and continued for the duration of bleeding. Tranexamic acid will reduce the menstrual blood flow but has no analgesic effect. Cyclical treatment with OCP is also effective but is not considered as the first line therapy, for heavy regular menstrual bleeding and dysmenorrhoea, as long treatment cycles are required.

Q. 7 (E)

Since this patient has heavy menstrual bleeding with regular 28-day cycles, without any structural lesions, tranexamic acid administered during each bleeding episode is the first line treatment, as it will reduce the blood loss. Cyclical treatment with norethisterone or OCP is also effective, but is not considered as the first line therapy, for heavy regular menstrual bleeding lesions, cyclical treatment is required. Dilatation and curettage is not necessary as she is under 40 years of age, has no risk factors for endometrial carcinoma and the transvaginal ultrasound scan is normal.

Q. 7a (D)

Since this patient has frequent irregular bleeding without any structural lesions, cyclical treatment with OCP or norethisterone will be effective. However, norethisterone is a better option as she is 36 years of age and is obese.

Q. 8 (D)

Polypectomy by hysterotomy or hysterectomy are major procedures and are not necessary, as the polyp can be successfully resected under direct vision by hysteroscopy. Endometrial ablation should not be done as it will preclude histological examination.

Q. 9 (A)

This woman who is anaemic due to severe bleeding responded to treatment with norethisterone, but symptoms recurred after cessation of treatment. No abnormalities are detected on the ultrasound scan and the histology is normal. Therefore, the best option is to insert a levonorgestrel-releasing intrauterine device, which would provide long-term treatment. Hysterectomy is also a suitable alternative if bleeding recurs, after inserting a levonorgestrel releasing intrauterine device. Endometrial ablation would be an option if she refuses hysterectomy.

Q. 9a (C)

This woman who is anaemic due to severe bleeding did not respond to treatment with norethisterone, even though no abnormalities are detected on the ultrasound scan and the histology is normal. Therefore, she may not respond to insertion of a levonorgestrel-releasing intrauterine device. Hysterectomy is a better option even though she does not have a structural lesion, as she is 44 years of age, has been having AUB for 6 months, is anaemic and failed to respond to medical treatment. Endometrial ablation would be an option if she refuses hysterectomy.

Q. 10. (D)

Since she has a symptomatic submucous fibroid causing heavy menstrual bleeding, surgical treatment is indicated. The best surgical option is hysteroscopic resection, because it is a small submucous fibroid less than 5 cm in diameter. If myomectomy is performed by laparoscopy or laparotomy, it is necessary to cut through the entire thickness of the myometrium, thereby increasing the risk of uterine rupture during subsequent deliveries.

Q. 11 (D)

This woman has large fibroids causing heavy menstrual bleeding with resultant anaemia. Even though she has only one child she is 43 years of age. Therefore, the best treatment option is hysterectomy with preservation of the ovaries, if they are normal. GnRH analogues could be given for three months prior to surgery, to reduce the size and the vascularity of the tumour, but it will not cause permanent relief of symptoms, as the fibroids are large and multiple. Hysterectomy is safer and offers a more complete cure than myomectomy and uterine artery embolization. The latter procedures are not indicated as she is more than 40 years of age.

Q. 12 (E)

The fibroid polyp can be removed vaginally after clamping and tying the pedicle. The pedicle of a large fibroid polyp is usually too thick to be twisted like in the case of a normal polypectomy, for the removal of a mucoid cervical polyp. Hysterectomy is not indicated as there are no other uterine fibroids. Uterine artery embolization is not used to treat fibroid polyps.

Q. 13 (A)

This patient has typical symptoms (menorrhagia and secondary dysmenorrhoea), signs (uniform enlargement of the uterus) and ultrasonic features (uniform uterine enlargement with myometrial thickening) of adenomyosis. The only effective treatment for adenomyosis is hysterectomy. Medical treatment is not very effective and is carried out only if the woman desires future fertility.

Q. 14 (B)

Total hysterectomy is the best treatment option because of the risk of underlying malignancy or progression to cancer. Since this woman is premenopausal removal of ovaries is optional and should be discussed with the woman. However, bilateral salpingectomy should be performed as it reduces the risk of future ovarian cancer. Routine lymphadenectomy has no benefit. Endometrial ablation is not recommended, because complete and persistent endometrial destruction cannot be ensured and intrauterine adhesion formation may preclude endometrial histological surveillance. Insertion of a LNGIUS is recommended, only if the woman strongly desires future fertility.

Q. 15 (D)

Q. 16 (B)

Explanation for questions 15 and 16

When uniform thickening of the endometrium is found on the ultrasound scan in a premenopausal woman, the next step is to perform an endometrial biopsy as an outpatient procedure. Direct visualisation of the endometrial cavity with a hysteroscope and biopsy of suspicious areas is recommended, if there is irregular or focal thickening of the endometrium, or if outpatient sampling fails, or is non-diagnostic. Use of MRI and CT scans are not recommended for diagnosis of endometrial hyperplasia.

REFERENCES

- Andrew M Kaunitz. Approach to abnormal uterine bleeding in non-pregnant reproductive-age women, up to date—August 2014.
- Malcolm G. Munro. FIGO classification system (PALM-COEIN) for causes of abnormal uterine bleeding in non-gravid women of reproductive age. International Journal of Gynaecology and Obstetrics-113 (2011).
- John W. Ely. Abnormal Uterine Bleeding: A Management Algorithm—The Journal of the American Board of Family Medicine.

2

Primary Amenorrhoea

Primary amenorrhoea is a condition in which a girl fails to menstruate by the age of 15 years. Investigations should be commenced if a girl fails to develop secondary sexual characteristics by the age of 13 years.

NORMAL PUBERTY

This is the time during which a girl becomes sexually mature and functionally able to reproduce. The changes which occur at puberty are the development of secondary sexual characteristics and onset of menstruation.

Secondary Sexual Characteristics

Development of axillary hair (13 yrs) and pubic hair (9 yrs).

Breast development (9 yrs).

The growth spurt (10–14 yrs).

SEXUAL DIFFERENTIATION IN UTERO

- The genetic sex at fertilisation can be XX or XY.
- The gonads develop very early in embryonic life.
- The testis functions during embryonic life.
- It produces müllerian inhibitory factor, which prevents the development of the müllerian system, which forms the uterus, tubes and upper two-thirds of the vagina and testosterone which causes masculinisation of the external genitalia.
- Therefore, a XY foetus will be born with male external and internal genitalia, only if the testis develops and functions during embryonic life.
- The development of the female internal and external genitalia is not under the influence of any hormones and the ovary does not produce any hormones *in utero*.
- Therefore, in the absence of a functioning testis *in utero*, a XY foetus will be born with female internal and external genitalia, the same as a XX foetus with or without an ovary.
- If the testicular function is impaired *in utero*, a XY foetus will have ambiguous external genitalia. The same will occur in a female foetus exposed to androgens *in utero*.

Menarche is the occurrence of the first menstrual period.

The occurrence of puberty and menarche requires the proper function of

- hypothalamus,
- pituitary,
- ovaries,
- uterus,
- and outflow tract

Failure of any one level will result in amenorrhoea.

CLINICAL PRESENTATION

A girl with primary amenorrhoea can present with:

- normal secondary sexual characteristics,
- absence of secondary sexual characteristics,
- virilising features.

CAUSES OF AMENORRHOEA IN A PATIENT WITH NORMAL SECONDARY SEXUAL CHARACTERISTICS

- Structural defects (XX)—
  - Imperforate hymen, vaginal septum
  - Absent vagina
  - Absent vagina and uterus—Mayer-Rokitansky-Küster-Hauser syndrome
- Constitutional delay (XX)
- Androgen insensitivity syndrome (XY)

Oestrogen should be present in these patients as this hormone is required for the development of secondary sexual characteristics. Therefore, except in testicular feminisation, all the other patients in this group have a functioning hypothalamic pituitary ovarian tract, with the ovary producing normal amounts of oestrogen and progesterone.

In androgen insensitivity syndrome (testicular feminisation syndrome) the patient is a male with normal amounts of testosterone, but its function is impaired due to a structural abnormality of the androgen receptors, due to an abnormality of the androgen receptor gene. In the absence of masculinising effects of testosterone, the testicular and adrenal oestrogens act unopposed to bring about good breast development. The effects of testosterone on the end organs are absent and the patient will have scanty axillary, pubic and body hair.

CAUSES OF AMENORRHOEA IN A PATIENT WITH ABSENT SECONDARY SEXUAL CHARACTERISTICS

- These patients do not have oestrogen, due to a failure at some point of the hypothalamic pituitary ovarian axis, resulting in failure of the ovary to produce oestrogen.
- Short stature will be present in those with empty sella syndrome, as growth hormone secretion is affected and in Turner syndrome, due to a genetic defect. The height will be normal in other patients.

HYPOGONADOTROPIC HYPOGONADISM

This condition is due to failure of the hypothalamus to secrete GnRH or failure of the pituitary to secrete FSH and LH.

Hypothalamic Causes (XX)

- Isolated GnRH deficiency—olfactogenital syndrome (Kallman syndrome)
- Excessive weight loss/anorexia nervosa
- Excessive exercise
- Psychological stresses

Isolated GnRH deficiency is due to maldevelopment of neurones in the arcuate nucleus of the hypothalamus. The pituitary is normal and can be stimulated with exogenous GnRH. The sense of smell is also absent. The other causes are acquired and are more often causes of secondary amenorrhoea.

Pituitary Causes (XX)

- Empty sella syndrome
- Tumours
- Surgery
- Irradiation

HYPERGONADOTROPIC AMENORRHOEA

- In these patients the function of the hypothalamus and the pituitary are normal but the ovary fails to respond to gonadotropins secreted by the pituitary.
- There will be a high level of gonadotropins due to failure of the negative feedback effect of ovarian hormones.
  - Gonadal agenesis (XX or XY)

    In these patients gonads fail to develop *in utero* in both XX and XY foetuses.

Therefore, XY foetuses will be born with female internal and external genitalia, same as XX foetuses.

- Gonadal dysgenesis—Turner syndrome (XO)
- Resistant ovary syndrome (XX)
- Premature ovarian failure (XX)

Causes of Amenorrhoea in those with Heterosexual Development

- Congenital adrenal hyperplasia (XX)
- Androgen secreting tumour (XX)
- True hermaphrodite (XX or XY)
- 5-alpha reductase deficiency (XY)
- Absent müllerian inhibitor (XY)

CLINICAL PRESENTATION OF PRIMARY AMENORRHOEA WITH NORMAL SECONDARY SEXUAL CHARACTERISTICS

Cryptomenorrhoea due to Imperforate Hymen/Transverse Vaginal Septum

Symptoms

- Present early by the age of 13–14 years.
- Monthly lower abdominal pain.
- Difficulty in passing urine/retention due to the haematocolpos.
- Continuous pain.

Signs

- An abdominal mass may be felt if a large haematocolpos is present.
- A bluish bulging hymenal membrane is seen, if there is an imperforate hymen.
- A haematocolpos can be felt on rectal examination.
- In the case of a vaginal septum the vagina appears to be blind ended, or there may appear to be a thick pink septum.

Cryptomenorrhoea due to Absent Vagina

- If the vagina is absent monthly abdominal pain may be present but the other symptoms may not be present as there is no haematocolpos.
- A large abdominal mass will not be felt as there is no haematocolpos.
- A smaller mass can be felt due to the haematometron.
- The vaginal area will appear as a dimple.

Absent Uterus and Vagina

- There will be no monthly abdominal pain, or an abdominal mass as there is no cryptomenorrhoea.
- The vaginal area will appear as a dimple.

Androgen Insensitivity Syndrome

- Secondary sexual characteristics will be present but axillary and pubic hair will be absent and body hair will be scanty.
- Breasts will be well developed.
- A short blind vagina will be present. The uterus and ovaries will be absent.
- The testis may be felt in the inguinal or pubic region.

Constitutional Delay

- There may be a family history of delayed menarche, or history of a serious childhood illness, or evidence of malnutrition.
- Early pubertal changes may be present and there will be no other abnormalities. External genitalia will be normal.

Investigations

Ultrasound scan is the first investigation which should be performed, in a patient with normal secondary sexual characteristics and primary amenorrhoea.

- If the uterus is present and there is evidence of cryptomenorrhoea, a diagnosis of outflow tract abnormality can be made.
- If the uterus is present and there is no evidence of cryptomenorrhoea, a diagnosis of delayed menarche is made.
- If the uterus is absent, the karyotype is done. If the karyotype is XX, the diagnosis is Mayer-Rokitansky syndrome.

- If the karyotype is XY, the diagnosis is testicular feminization. Serum testosterone levels and gonadal biopsy can be done to confirm the diagnosis.

Treatment

The aim of treatment of primary amenorrhoea is to restore:
- secondary sexual characteristics,
- menstruation,
- fertility,
- sexual function.

In this group of patients secondary sexual characteristics are present and the aim is to restore the other functions.

Imperforate Hymen XX

- A cruciate incision of the hymen is performed and the blood is allowed to drain.
- A drain is not inserted because of the risk of introducing infection.
- Antibiotics are given.
- Menstruation will be restored from the next month.
- Sexual activity will be normal.
- Fertility is not affected.

Vaginal Septum XX

- Excision and reconstruction is more difficult than in the case of an imperforate hymen.
- If surgery is successful, cure will be complete with restoration of menstruation, sexual activity and fertility.

Absent Vagina XX

- The best treatment option is to reconstruct a vagina which communicates with the uterus.
- If surgery is successful, the cure will be complete with restoration of menstruation, sexual activity and fertility.
- A hysterectomy may be needed later to relieve symptoms if surgery is not successful. Also a vagina suitable for sexual intercourse may have to be constructed at the appropriate time

- Continuous administration of oral contraceptive pills, or 3 monthly injections of depot medroxyprogesterone acetate, can be used temporarily to suppress menstruation.

Absent Uterus and Vagina XX

- Reconstruct a vagina suitable for sexual intercourse at an appropriate time.
- Fertility and menstruation cannot be restored.

Androgen Insensitivity Syndrome XY

- The cloacal vagina may be adequate for intercourse or an artificial vagina can be constructed.
- Menstruation cannot be restored as there is no uterus and an outflow tract.
- Fertility cannot be restored.
- The gonads should be removed after secondary sexual characteristics are well developed, as a dysgerminoma can occur in these abnormal gonads.

Delayed Puberty XX

Observe for 6 months.

CLINICAL PRESENTATION OF PRIMARY AMENORRHOEA WITH ABSENT SECONDARY SEXUAL CHARACTERISTICS

Clinical Presentation

- The patient will present with failure to attain menarche and failure to develop secondary sexual characteristics.
- Short stature will occur if growth hormone secretion is affected (pituitary dwarfism) and in Turner syndrome.
- In Turner syndrome other stigmata such as webbing of the neck, increased carrying angle and wide spaced nipples may be present.
- In hypogonadotropic patients due to hypothalamic causes there may be a history of excessive exercise, loss of weight or psychological problems.

- If the lesion is in the pituitary, other pituitary hormones may also be absent and the patient can present with hypothyroidism or hypoadrenalism.

Investigations

- In patients without secondary sexual characteristics the problem is in the hypothalamic pituitary ovarian axis.
- Therefore, the first investigation is a hormone profile to determine the site of the lesion. FSH, LH and prolactin levels are done.
- If the FSH and LH levels are low, the lesion is in the hypothalamus or the pituitary.
- GnRH levels and other pituitary hormones should be estimated, to determine the exact site and extent of the lesion.
- In cases where the cause is in the hypothalamus or pituitary (hypogonadotropic) or if the prolactin levels are elevated, CT/MRI scans should be done, to exclude tumours or other intracranial lesions.
- If the FSH and LH levels are high, the lesion is in the ovary. A karyotype should be done to exclude Turner syndrome or XY gonadal agenesis.

MANAGEMENT

Hypogonadotropic Hypogonadism

- If gonadotropins are low and the patient is of normal height, the diagnosis is hypogonadotropic hypogonadism.
- If the lesion is in the hypothalamus, causative factors should be eliminated. Excessive exercise should be stopped. Anorexia nervosa and other psychological problems should be treated. Excessive weight gain or weight loss should be treated.
- In cases of isolated GnRH deficiency, GnRH can be administered in a pulsatile manner.
- If the condition is in the pituitary, it can be cured by administration of exogenous gonadotropins.

- If other pituitary hormones are involved, replacement should be done. Replacement therapy is theoretically possible in congenital pan hypopituitarism. Treatment is commenced with ACTH followed by TSH and later gonadotropins.
- Treatment will result in development of secondary sexual characteristics and menstruation. Ovulation induction at the appropriate time may restore fertility. Sexual function is possible as a normal vagina is present.
- An intracranial lesion should be excluded in all patients. Visual fields should be tested and CT and MRI scans should be done. If a tumour is present, surgery is needed.

Hypergonadotropic Hypogonadism

- In hypergonadotropic hypogonadism the ovaries are resistant to stimulation by gonadotropins.
- In Turner syndrome, resistant ovary syndrome, premature ovarian failure and gonadal agenesis (gonads are absent) restoration of fertility is not possible.
- Secondary sexual characteristics and menstruation can be induced by giving oestrogen alone for one year followed by long-term treatment with oestrogen and progesterone. Prolonged treatment with oestrogen alone can cause endometrial carcinoma if the uterus is present.
- Sexual activity is possible because a normal vagina is present.

INVESTIGATION OF HETEROSEXUAL PATIENTS

- The individual can be a male or a female
- The first step is to perform a karyotype.
- If the karyotype is XX, the individual is a female. The possibility of congenital adrenal hyperplasia, an androgen secreting ovarian tumour or an adrenal tumour should be suspected. If the virilisation is mild pre pubertal polycystic ovarian syndrome is a possibility.

- If the patient is a female, the next step is to perform serum 17-hydroxyprogesterone levels.
- If 17-hydroxyprogesterone is elevated, diagnosis of congenital adrenal hyperplasia is confirmed. Serum electrolytes should be done to exclude salt loss.
- Treatment with a large dose of glucocorticoids is commenced. Salt loss is corrected if present.
- Secondary sexual characteristics will develop and menstruation will occur.
- Fertility can be eventually restored after ovulation induction.
- Corrective surgery is done to reduce the size of the clitoris and to divide labial folds.

- In androgen secreting tumours serum testosterone will be very high. The diagnosis is confirmed by ultrasound scanning. Treatment is by surgical removal.
- If the karyotype is XY it is better to continue as a female as male sexual functions cannot be restored. The gonads should be removed to prevent further secretion of androgens and malignant transformation. Corrective surgery and cosmetic therapy is done for virilisation. Female secondary sexual characteristics can be induced with oestrogen alone if the uterus is absent. The cloacal vagina may be sufficient for sexual intercourse or a vagina can be reconstructed at the appropriate time. Fertility and menstruation cannot be restored.

QUESTIONS

1. A 15-year-old girl complains of failure to attain menarche. Her height is 4 feet. She has not yet developed secondary sexual characteristics.

   What is the next step in making a diagnosis?

   A. Perform a CT brain.

   B. Perform a hormone profile.

   C. Perform a karyotype.

   D. Perform an ultrasound scan.

   E. Perform laparoscopy and gonadal biopsy.

2. A 15-year-old girl complains of failure to attain menarche. Her height is 4 feet. She has not yet developed secondary sexual characteristics. Ultrasound scan reveals the presence of the uterus and vagina. The FSH and LH levels are high.

   What is the most likely diagnosis?

   A. Delayed menarche.

   B. Gonadal agenesis.

   C. Kallman's syndrome.

   D. Resistant ovary syndrome.

   E. Turner syndrome.

3. A 15-year-old girl complains of failure to attain menarche. Her height is 4 feet. She has not yet developed secondary sexual characteristics. Ultrasound scan reveals the presence of the uterus and vagina. The FSH and LH levels are high.

   What is the next step in confirming the diagnosis?

   A. Perform laparoscopy and gonadal biopsy.

   B. Perform a buccal smear.

   C. Perform a karyotype.

   D. Perform an examination under anaesthesia.

   E. Perform progesterone withdrawal test.

4. A 20-year-old girl complains of failure to attain menarche. She has not developed secondary sexual characteristics. The FSH and LH levels are high. The karyotype is XO.

Which of the following is the first step in the management?

A. Long-term cyclical oestrogen therapy.

B. Reassurance and explanation.

C. Removal of the streak gonads.

D. Treatment with growth hormone for 6 months.

E. Treatment with combined oral contraceptive pills.

4a. A 20-year-old girl complains of failure to attain menarche. She has not developed secondary sexual characteristics. The FSH and LH levels are high. The karyotype is XO.

Which of the following is the best treatment option?

A. Long-term treatment with oestrogen.

B. Reconstruction of an artificial vagina.

C. Removal of the streak gonads.

D. Treatment with growth hormone for 6 months.

E. Treatment with oestrogen for 1 year and maintenance with oestrogen and progesterone.

5. A 20-year-old girl complains of failure to attain menarche. She has not developed secondary sexual characteristics. Ultrasound scan reveals the presence of the uterus and vagina. The FSH and LH levels are high. The karyotype is XO.

Which of the following cannot be restored by treatment?

A. A slight increase in height.

B. Fertility.

C. Menstruation.

D. Secondary sexual characteristics.

E. Sexual activity.

6. A 16-year-old girl presents with primary amenorrhoea. Her height is 5 feet. She has no secondary sexual characteristics. Ultrasound scan reveals the presence of the uterus and vagina. She has high FSH and LH levels with low oestrogen levels. Karyotype is XY.

What is the most appropriate diagnosis?

A. Absence of müllerian inhibition.

B. Androgen insensitivity syndrome.

C. Gonadal agenesis.

D. Premature menopause

E. Turner syndrome.

7. A 16-year-old girl presents with primary amenorrhoea. Her height is 150 cm. She has no secondary sexual characteristics. Examination reveals the presence of the uterus and vagina. She has high FSH and LH levels with low oestrogen levels. Karyotype is XY.

What is the best treatment option for this patient?

A. Cosmetic therapy for hirsutism.

B. Restore fertility by treatment with GNRH analogues for 1 year followed by ovulation induction.

C. Restore secondary sexual characteristics and menstruation with oestrogen therapy for 1 year, followed by long-term oestrogen and progestogen therapy.

D. Restore secondary sexual characteristics and menstruation by long-term cyclical oestrogen therapy.

E. Treat with GNRH analogues for 1 year and follow up with long-term cyclical oestrogen and progestogen therapy.

8. A 20-year-old girl presents with primary amenorrhoea. She has good secondary sexual characteristics. The height is 152 cm. She has scanty axillary, pubic and body hair. Clinical examination and ultrasound scanning reveal a short blind vagina and absent uterus.

What is the most likely diagnosis?

A. Androgen insensitivity syndrome.

B. Gonadal dysgenesis.

C. Imperforate hymen.

D. Mayer-Rokitansky-Küster-Hauser syndrome

E. True hermaphrodite.

9. A 20-year-old girl presents with primary amenorrhoea. She has good secondary sexual characteristics. The height is 153 cm. She has scanty axillary, pubic and body hair. Clinical examination and ultrasound scanning reveal a short blind vagina and absent uterus.

What is the next step to establish the diagnosis?

A. Estimate pituitary gonadotropin levels.

B. Estimate serum testosterone levels.

C. Perform a buccal smear.

D. Perform a karyotype.

E. Perform laparoscopy and gonadal biopsy.

10. An 18-year-old girl presents with primary amenorrhoea. She has good secondary sexual characteristics. The height is 150 cm. She has scanty axillary, pubic and body hair. Clinical examination and ultrasound scanning reveal a short blind vagina and absent uterus. The karyotype is XY.

What is the most appropriate treatment option?

A. Cyclical treatment with combined oral contraceptive pills.

B. Hormone replacement therapy with oestrogen.

C. Reassurance and explanation only.

D. Reassurance, explanation and removal of the gonads.

E. Reconstruction of an artificial vagina.

11. A 14-year-old girl presents with primary amenorrhoea and monthly lower abdominal pain. She has good secondary sexual characteristics with axillary and pubic hair. Examination of the external genitalia reveals a bulging bluish membrane with no hymenal orifice.

What is the most appropriate next step required to arrive at a diagnosis?

A. Perform a hormone profile.

B. Perform a karyotype.

C. Perform a laparoscopy.

D. Perform a MRI scan.

E. Perform an ultrasound scan.

12. A 14-year-old girl presents with primary amenorrhoea and monthly lower abdominal pain. She has good secondary sexual characteristics with axillary and pubic hair. Examination of the external genitalia reveals a bulging bluish membrane with no hymenal orifice. Ultrasound scan reveals a haematocolpos.

What is the best treatment option?

A. Creation of a small hole in the hymenal membrane.

B. Cruciate incision in the hymenal membrane and insertion of a drain for a week.

C. Cruciate incision in the hymenal membrane.

D. Excision of the hymen.

E. Vaginal repair.

13. A 16-year-old girl presents with primary amenorrhoea and monthly abdominal pain. She has good secondary sexual characteristics with axillary and pubic hair. Abdominal examination reveals a firm, tender, abdomino-pelvic mass corresponding in size to a 14 weeks pregnant uterus. Examination of the external genitalia reveals absence of the vagina.

What is the next investigation you would carry out?

A. Perform a karyotype.

B. Perform a laparoscopy.

C. Perform a MRI scan.

D. Perform a pelvic examination under anaesthesia

E. Perform an ultrasound scan.

14. A 16-year-old girl presents with primary amenorrhoea and monthly lower abdominal pain. She has good secondary sexual characteristics with axillary and pubic hair. Examination of

the external genitalia reveals absence of the vagina. Ultrasound scan reveals a haematometron.

What is the best treatment option?

A. Continuous treatment with oral contraceptive pills.

B. Excision of the hymen.

C. Injection of depot medroxyprogesterone acetate once in three months.

D. Perform a hysterectomy.

E. Surgical creation of a vagina which communicates with the uterus.

15. A 16-year-old girl presents with primary amenorrhoea. She has good secondary sexual characteristics with axillary and pubic hair. Examination of the external genitalia reveals absence of the vagina. Ultrasound scan reveals absence of the uterus.

    What is the most likely diagnosis?

    A. Androgen insensitivity syndrome.

    B. Gonadal agenesis.

    C. Congenital adrenal hyperplasia.

    D. Mayer-Rokitansky-Küster-Hauser syndrome.

    E. True hermaphrodite.

16. A 16-year-old girl presents with primary amenorrhoea. She has good secondary sexual characteristics with axillary and pubic hair. Examination of the external genitalia reveals absence of the vagina. Ultrasound scan reveals absence of the uterus.

    What is the most appropriate investigation to confirm the diagnosis?

    A. Perform a buccal smear.

    B. Perform a hormone profile.

    C. Perform a karyotype.

    D. Perform a laparoscopy and gonadal biopsy.

    E. Perform a MRI scan.

17. A 20-year-old married woman presents with primary amenorrhoea and inability to perform sexual intercourse. A diagnosis of Mayer-Rokitansky-Küster-Hauser syndrome is made.

    What is the most appropriate management?

    A. Dilatation of the vaginal dimple

    B. *In vitro* fertilisation.

    C. Long-term treatment with oestrogen.

    D. Long-term treatment with oral contraceptive pills.

    E. Surgical creation of a vagina suitable for sexual intercourse.

18. An infant is found to have clitoral enlargement and some degree of labial fusion.

    What is the first step in arriving at a diagnosis?

    A. Perform a karyotype.

    B. Perform an ultrasound scan.

    C. Perform blood 17-hydroxyprogesterone levels.

    D. Perform serum 5α-reductase levels.

    E. Perform serum testosterone levels.

19. An infant is found to have clitoral enlargement and some degree of labial fusion. The karyotype is XX.

    What is the next step in arriving at a diagnosis?

    A. Perform 5α-reductase levels.

    B. Perform an ultrasound scan.

    C. Perform blood 17-hydroxyprogesterone levels.

    D. Perform serum cortisol levels.

    E. Perform serum testosterone levels.

20. A 2-year-old child is found to have hirsutism clitoral enlargement and some degree of labial fusion. The karyotype is XX. Serum 17-hydroxyprogesterone levels are high.

    What is the most appropriate first step in the management?

A. Commence treatment with cortisol after puberty.

B. Commence treatment with gluco-corticoids

C. Cosmetic therapy for hirsutism.

D. Give a high salt diet.

E. Perform surgery to remove the tumour.

21. **A 13-year-old child, who is reared as a female, presents with hirsutism and deepening of the voice. The karyotype is XY. On examination there is hirsutism, partial fusion of the labia and clitoromegaly. Gonads could be felt in the inguinal region.**

    What is the most appropriate first step in the management?

    A. Commence cosmetic therapy for hirsutism and clitoromegaly.

    B. Perform surgery to remove the abnormal gonads.

    C. Rear the child as a male.

    D. Treat with oestrogen and progestogen.

    E. Treat with oestrogen.

22. **A 13-year-old child, who is reared as a female, presents with hirsutism and deepening of the voice. The karyotype is XY. On examination there is**

hirsutism, partial fusion of the labia and clitoromegaly. Gonads could be felt in the inguinal region. Surgery is performed to remove the abnormal gonads.

What is the most appropriate long-term management?

A. Commence cosmetic therapy for hirsutism and clitoromegaly.

B. Rear the child as a female.

C. Rear the child as a male.

D. Treat with oestrogen and progestogen.

E. Treat with oestrogen.

23. **A 15-year-old girl complains of failure to attain menarche. Her height is 5 feet. She has not yet developed secondary sexual characteristics. The FSH and LH levels are low.**

    What is the next step in confirming the diagnosis?

    A. Perform a buccal smear.

    B. Perform a karyotype.

    C. Perform a MRI scan.

    D. Perform an ultrasound scan.

    E. Perform GnRH and other pituitary hormone levels.

ANSWERS AND EXPLANATIONS

Q. 1 (B)

Failure to develop secondary sexual characteristics indicate failure of ovarian function which could be due to the absence of pituitary gonadotropins or ovarian failure. A hormone profile should be performed first to determine whether the abnormality is in the hypothalamus/pituitary or the ovary.

If the gonadotropins are low the lesion is in the hypothalamus or pituitary. Other pituitary hormone levels should be assayed to exclude an empty sella syndrome/pan hypopituitarism as she is

short. A CT scan of the brain should be performed if a hypothalamic or pituitary cause is suspected to exclude a tumour.

If the gonadotropins are high the cause is ovarian failure. Because the patient is short a karyotype should be performed next to confirm Turner syndrome. Ultrasound scanning, Laparoscopy and gonadal biopsy could be performed later but may not be necessary to establish a diagnosis.

Q. 2 (E)

As the gonadotropin levels are high the cause is ovarian failure and the most likely causes are Gonadal agenesis, resistant ovary syndrome or Turner syndrome. Because this patient is short the most likely diagnosis is Turner syndrome. In gonadal agenesis and resistant ovary syndrome the patient will be of normal height.

In delayed menarche the gonadotropins will be in the low normal range. In Kallmann's syndrome the gonadotropins will be low.

Q. 3 (C)

Failure to develop secondary sexual characteristics indicates failure of ovarian function which could be due to the absence of pituitary gonadotropins or ovarian failure. High FSH and LH levels indicate ovarian failure. Since the patient is short the most likely cause is Turner syndrome. Therefore, the next step in the diagnosis is to perform a karyotype to confirm Turner syndrome. In Turner syndrome the karyotype will be XO or a mosaic of XO. Laparoscopy and gonadal biopsy could be performed later but is not necessary to establish a diagnosis. Progesterone withdrawal test will not be positive as there is no oestrogen in the circulation.

Q. 4 (B)

Q. 4a (E)

Q. 5 (B)

Explanation for questions 4, 4a and 5

A complete cure in cases of primary amenorrhoea requires restoration of menstruation, secondary sexual characteristics, sexual activity and fertility.

This patient has Turner syndrome. Normal sexual intercourse is possible because the vagina is present. Fertility cannot be restored because there is no treatment available to induce streak ovaries to produce an ovum. *In vitro* fertilisation is a difficult option because it needs ovum donation and administration of a large amount of ovarian hormones. She is short due to a defect in the chromosomes and the height cannot be restored by treatment with growth hormone.

The first step in the management of all cases of primary amenorrhoea is reassurance and explanation of the condition, the treatment options and the results which can be achieved by treatment. The patient and the parents should understand the future prospects.

The best treatment option is to give oestrogen for one year, followed by long-term treatment with oestrogen and progesterone. This will result in monthly withdrawal bleeding, some amount of breast development and a slight increase in height. Sexual activity is normal since the vagina is present.

Q. 6 (C)

The karyotype can be XY in androgen insensitivity syndrome, gonadal agenesis and absence of müllerian inhibition. In androgen insensitivity syndrome female secondary sexual characteristics will be present. If the patient is a genetic male with absent müllerian inhibitory factor, testosterone will be present and she should be virilised. Therefore, the most likely diagnosis is gonadal agenesis. In these patients the genetic sex could be XX or XY, but the gonads fail to develop. Since there is no testosterone and müllerian inhibitory factor *in utero*, a XY foetus will be born with female external and internal genitalia. Since gonads are absent the apparent female will not have testosterone or oestrogen. Hence "she" will not develop female secondary sexual characteristics or menstruation at puberty and will not be virilised, even though the karyotype is XY. The FSH and LH levels will be high due to absence of the negative feedback effect of gonadal hormones. In premature menopause and Turner syndrome FSH and LH levels will be high, but the karyotype is XX in the former and XO in the latter. The uterus and vagina will be absent only in androgen insensitivity syndrome.

Q. 7 (C)

Since the karyotype is XY and the patient has female external and internal genitalia and amenorrhoea, with no male or female secondary sexual characteristics the diagnosis is gonadal agenesis. Even though "she" is a genetic male the gonads have failed to develop *in utero*. Even though this patient is a genetic male "she" has to be reared as a female as "she" has normal female external genitalia.

Fertility cannot be restored as there is no ovary to produce ova. Treatment with GnRH analogues is useless as there is no ovary which can be stimulated by gonadotropins. Therefore, the best and only treatment option is to restore secondary sexual characteristics and menstruation by oestrogen therapy for 6 months, followed by long-term oestrogen and progesterone therapy. These effects can be obtained by cyclical oestrogen therapy alone, but since a uterus is present "she" could later develop an endometrial carcinoma, due to prolonged unopposed oestrogen therapy. Since there is no testis to produce testosterone "she" will not be virilised and does not need cosmetic therapy for hirsutism. Normal female sexual functions are present.

Q. 8 (A)

The most appropriate diagnosis is androgen insensitivity syndrome (testicular feminisation). In testicular feminisation the patient is a genetic male with functioning testes, which produce testosterone and müllerian inhibitory factor *in utero*. Therefore, the uterus and the upper two thirds of the vagina will be absent. The function of testosterone is impaired, due to a structural abnormality of the androgen receptors, due to an abnormality of the androgen receptor gene. Therefore, the testicular and adrenal oestrogens act unopposed to bring about good breast development. The masculinising effects of testosterone are absent and the patient will have scanty axillary, pubic and body hair.

The closest differential diagnosis is Mayer-Rokitansky syndrome in which the uterus and vagina will be absent, but secondary sexual characteristics will be present as the hypothalamus, pituitary and ovaries are normal. The karyotype will be XX and she will have normal axillary, pubic and body hair.

In gonadal dysgenesis and Kallman's syndrome secondary sexual characteristics will be absent due to ovarian failure in the former and absence of pituitary gonadotropins in the latter. Virilisation will occur in a true hermaphrodite as the testes are present.

Q. 9 (D)

The diagnosis most probably is androgen insensitivity syndrome because her height is normal and she has good female secondary sexual characteristics, with scanty body hair and absent vagina and uterus. The next step is to perform a karyotype. The diagnosis can be established if the karyotype is XY. Estimation of serum testosterone levels and gonadal biopsy may be done later, but is not essential for initial diagnostic purposes. The diagnosis can be confirmed by the clinical picture and the XY genotype.

Q. 10 (D)

The diagnosis is androgen insensitivity syndrome because the karyotype is XY, her height is normal and she has good female secondary sexual characteristics, with scanty body hair and absent vagina and uterus.

Cyclical treatment with combined oral contraceptive pills or hormone replacement therapy with oestrogen is not indicated, as she has good secondary sexual characteristics, due to the unopposed action of adrenal and testicular oestrogens. Moreover, it is not possible to induce menstruation as she does not have a uterus. Vaginal repair may not be necessary, as the blind ending cloacal vagina is usually adequate for sexual intercourse. Fertility cannot be restored as there is no uterus or ovaries. She has to be reared as a female as she has female secondary sexual characteristics and female external genitalia. Reassurance and explanation is essential as she should understand her future prospects. The abnormal testes can undergo malignant change. Therefore, the testes should be removed after the development of secondary sexual characteristics because testicular oestrogen plays a role in their development. This is usually done at about 14 years of age.

Q. 11 (E)

This patient has an imperforate hymen because she has monthly lower abdominal pain, good secondary sexual characteristics and a bulging bluish hymenal membrane, due to the collection of blood in the vagina. The most appropriate next step is to perform an ultrasound scan to confirm the presence of the uterus, ovaries and vagina and a haematocolpos. No other investigations are needed as the diagnosis can be confirmed by the clinical picture and ultrasound scanning.

Q. 12 (C)

This patient has an imperforate hymen because she has monthly lower abdominal pain, good secondary sexual characteristics, a bulging bluish hymenal membrane due to the collection of blood in the vagina and a haematocolpos is seen on the scan. The best and only treatment option is to make a cruciate incision in the hymenal membrane and to allow the blood to drain gradually. A drain should not be inserted because of the risk of introducing infection. Normal menstruation will occur from the next month. Fertility and sexual function will be normal.

Q. 13 (E)

This patient most probably has crypto-menorrhoea because she has primary amenorrhoea, monthly lower abdominal pain, good secondary sexual characteristics, a tender abdomino pelvic mass and absence of the vagina. She most probably has a haematometron. The next step in the management is to perform an ultrasound scan to confirm the haematometron and absence of the vagina. It is essential to exclude abnormalities of the renal system as these can co-exist.

Q. 14 (E)

This patient most probably has crypto-menorrhoea with a haematometron, because she has primary amenorrhoea, monthly lower abdominal pain, good secondary sexual characteristics, a tender abdomino-pelvic mass and absence of the vagina. The diagnosis is confirmed by the presence of a haematometron on the ultrasound scan. The best treatment option is surgical creation of a vagina which communicates with the uterus. This operation is a difficult procedure with low success rates. However, good results can be obtained in specialised centres. If the operation is successful, monthly menstruation, sexual activity and fertility can be restored. If the operation is not successful, menstruation will have to be stopped, by giving OCP continuously or with DMPA injections. A hysterectomy may be necessary as an ultimate measure. A vagina which is suitable for sexual intercourse can be constructed surgically at the appropriate time. Menstruation and fertility cannot be restored in these patients.

Q. 15 (D)

The probable diagnosis is Mayer-Roki-tansky syndrome, as the uterus and vagina are absent, body hair is normal and secondary sexual characteristics are present, indicating normal function of the hypothalamus, pituitary and ovaries. The closest differential diagnosis is testicular feminisation, as she has good secondary sexual characteristics, with absence of the uterus and vagina. However, the body hair will be scanty in this condition. In congenital adrenal hyperplasia the patient will be virilised and the uterus and the vagina will be present. In gonadal agenesis secondary sexual characteristics will be absent, due to absence of the ovaries. Virilisation will occur in a true hermaphrodite, as the testes are present.

Q. 16 (C)

The probable diagnosis is Mayer-Rokitansky syndrome, as the uterus and vagina are absent, body hair is normal and secondary sexual characteristics are present, indicating normal function of the hypothalamus, pituitary and ovaries. The diagnosis can be confirmed if the karyotype is XX. The closest differential diagnosis is testicular feminisation syndrome, where the karyotype will be XY. A laparoscopy and gonadal biopsy may be performed later but is not essential to confirm the diagnosis.

Q. 17 (E)

The most appropriate treatment of this condition is to restore sexual function by creating a vagina suitable for sexual intercourse. A vaginal dimple may be present, but it may be too shallow for dilatation to be successful. Since the uterus is absent *in vitro* fertilisation is not feasible. Treatment with oestrogen or OCP has no benefits as secondary sexual characteristics are present in this condition and it is not possible to restore menstruation as the uterus is absent.

Q. 18 (A)

A child born with ambiguous external genitalia could be a female who has been exposed to androgens, such as in the case of congenital adrenal hyperplasia, or a true hermaphrodite, or an under masculinised male. Such a male could have 5α-reductase deficiency, or abnormal androgen receptors, or müllerian inhibitor deficiency. Therefore, the first step in the diagnosis is to perform a karyotype, to diagnose whether the child is a male or a female, because further investigations would depend on the genetic sex. However, a true hermaphrodite could be XX or XY.

Q. 19 (C)

As the karyotype is XX the child is a female. The child has been exposed to androgens *in utero* from the mother or the child has congenital adrenal hyperplasia. The rare possibility of a true hermaphrodite with a XX karyotype should also be considered. The next step is to perform blood 17-hydroxyprogesterone levels, to confirm/exclude congenital adrenal hyperplasia, which is a treatable condition. An ultrasound scan should be performed next, because the uterus ovaries and vagina are present in congenital adrenal hyperplasia.

Q. 20 (B)

A diagnosis of congenital adrenal hyperplasia can be made because the karyotype is XX and there is hirsutism, labial fusion and elevation of 17-hydroxyprogesterone. The first step in the management is to commence treatment with a large dose of corticosteroids to suppress the adrenal function. Treatment should be commenced immediately to prevent the harmful effects of excessive adrenal function. All female functions will be restored in due course. Cosmetic treatment will be required for hirsutism and clitoromegaly. Salt loss should be prevented.

Q. 21 (B) and Q. 22 (B)

Since the karyotype is XY with ambiguous external genitalia this child is a male with impaired testicular function. The child should continue to be reared as a female as male sexual functions cannot be restored.

The first step is to remove the gonads to prevent further secretion of androgens and malignant transformation. Corrective surgery and cosmetic therapy should be done for virilisation. Female secondary sexual characteristics can be induced with oestrogen alone as the uterus is absent. The cloacal vagina may be sufficient for sexual intercourse or a vagina can be reconstructed at the appropriate time. Fertility and menstruation cannot be restored.

Q. 23 (E)

Since FSH and LH levels are low the lesion is in the hypothalamus or the pituitary. The next step is to perform GnRH levels and the pituitary hormone levels to determine the site and the extent of the lesion. A CT/ MRI scan should be performed next to exclude an intracranial tumour. In cases of isolated GnRH deficiency, GnRH can be administered in a pulsatile manner.

If the condition is in the pituitary, it can be cured by administration of exogenous gonadotropins.

If other pituitary hormones are involved replacement should be done. Replacement therapy is theoretically possible in congenital panhypopituitarism. Treatment is commenced with ACTH followed by TSH and later gonadotropins.

3

Secondary Amenorrhoea

Secondary amenorrhoea is cessation of menstruation for six continuous months, in a woman who has previously had regular monthly periods.

CAUSES

- Physiological causes
  - Pregnancy
  - Lactation
  - Menopause
- Hypothalamic causes
  - Excessive weight loss/anorexia nervosa
  - Excessive exercise
  - Psychological stress
  - Head injuries
- Pituitary causes
  - Sheehan's syndrome
  - Hyperprolactinaemia—micro and macro adenomas
  - Irradiation
  - Head injuries
- Ovarian causes
  - Polycystic ovarian syndrome (PCOS)
  - Premature ovarian failure—genetic or autoimmune
  - Irradiation
  - Chemotherapy
  - Androgen or oestrogen secreting tumours

- Uterine causes
  - Asherman's syndrome
  - Cervical stenosis
- Systemic causes
  - Chronic debilitating illnesses
  - Weight loss
  - Other endocrine diseases—thyroid, adrenal
- Drugs
  - Depot medroxyprogesterone acetate injections
  - Progesterone implants
  - Levonorgestrel-releasing intrauterine device
  - Oral contraceptive pills
  - Antidepressant drugs

DIAGNOSIS

History

- Exclude pregnancy
- Weight gain—PCOS, Cushing's syndrome
- Weight loss—Anorexia nervosa
- Hirsutism—PCOS, androgen secreting ovarian tumours
- Excessive exercise
- Psychological stresses
- Hot flushes—premature ovarian failure
- Radiotherapy, chemotherapy
- Headache, visual disturbances—intracranial lesion

- Galactorrhoea—pituitary macro/micro adenoma
- Severe postpartum haemorrhage and failure of lactation—Sheehan's syndrome
- Vigorous uterine curettage, especially postpartum for retained placental tissue—Asherman's syndrome.
- Surgery of the cervix or cervical tears at delivery—cervical stenosis
- Drugs—hormonal contraceptives, psychiatric drugs, performance enhancing drugs.
- Chronic illnesses—tuberculosis
- Premature ovarian failure—family history, history of autoimmune disease, occurrence of hot flashes

Examination

- Increased BMI in PCOS and Cushing's syndrome.
- Low BMI in excessive exercise and anorexia nervosa.
- Mild hirsutism, acne, obesity and acanthosis nigricans in PCOS.
- Gross hirsutism, clitoromegaly and voice changes in testosterone secreting ovarian or adrenal tumours.
- Truncal obesity, moon face, striae and easy bruising in Cushing's syndrome.
- Thyroid enlargement with signs of hyper/hypothyroidism.
- Bi-temporal hemianopia and neurological signs in pituitary tumours.
- Breast secretions especially in a nulliparous woman indicate hyperprolactinaemia.

Investigations

- Transvaginal ultrasound scan to detect:
  - cryptomenorrhoea due to cervical stenosis,
  - polycystic ovarian syndrome,
  - intrauterine adhesions in Asherman's syndrome.
- Full blood count, ESR.
- Hormone levels
  - Elevated FSH and LH:

Both are (FSH > than 40 IU/L) elevated in ovarian failure. In PCOS LH is elevated and the FSH:LH ratio is changed.
  - Low FSH and LH:

Low levels are found in failure at the level of the hypothalamus or pituitary. It is difficult to determine the exact aetiology. Clinical symptoms and signs may be helpful.
  - Increased prolactin:

If the level is greater than 1000 mIU/L, a pituitary tumour is suspected. Lower levels will occur in PCOS. Blood should not be taken soon after breast examination.
  - Mild elevation of testosterone

Occur in PCOS.
  - Gross elevation of testosterone:

Occur in androgen secreting tumours.
  - Thyroid hormones.
  - Cortisol is elevated in Cushing's syndrome.
  - If all pituitary hormones are depressed Sheehan's syndrome is suspected.
- CT scan of the brain should be performed if an intracranial lesion is suspected.

ASHERMAN'S SYNDROME

- Occurs if the basal layer of the endometrium is damaged by vigorous curettage.
- More common after puerperal curettage in secondary postpartum haemorrhage, because of the presence of infection. Low oestrogen level during lactation will also favour adhesion formation.
- Diagnosis is suspected by the history. Adhesions could be seen by performing a transvaginal scan or a hysterosalpingogram. The diagnosis is confirmed by hysteroscopy.
- Treatment is hysteroscopy and adhesiolysis with a curette.
- An IUCD is inserted to prevent reformation of adhesions.

Cervical Stenosis

- Is suspected if there is a history of surgery of the cervix or cervical tears at delivery.
- Diagnosed by visualizing a haematometron by ultrasound scanning.
- The cervix is dilated and collected blood is allowed to drain.

Premature Ovarian Failure

- A family history may be present.
- Is diagnosed if FSH levels are high. Two tests should be done 6 weeks apart.
- An auto-antibody level should be done.
- A karyotype is done to exclude a Turner mosaic.
- Treatment is by hormone replacement therapy. Ovaries cannot be stimulated to function again.

Pituitary Tumours

- Suspected if the prolactin level is greater than 1000 mIU /L.
- Confirmed by CT/ MRI scan.
- Pituitary macroadenomas require surgery.
- Microadenomas can be treated with bromocriptine or cabergoline.

Hypopituitarism (Sheehan Syndrome)

- Is suspected if there is a history of post-partum haemorrhage and failure of lactation.
- Symptoms of hypothyroidism and adrenal failure may be present.
- Thyroid, adrenal and pituitary hormones will be low.
- Treated by first replacing corticosteroids and thyroxine. Ovulation induction is carried out with gonadotropin injections if pregnancy is desired.

Hypothalamic Causes

- Treat weight loss, obesity, psychiatric illnesses, chronic illnesses and avoid excessive exercise.
- Reassurance and explanation is essential in these cases.

Drug Induced Amenorrhoea

- Use of hormonal contraceptives should be stopped. An intrauterine contraceptive device can be used.
- Other drugs should be reduced if possible.

Ovarian and Adrenal Tumours

- Should be surgically removed.

Polycystic Ovarian Syndrome

- PCOS is a syndrome which causes ovarian dysfunction. It has the cardinal features of hyperandrogenism and polycystic ovarian morphology.
- The ovarian androgen production is increased, due partly to disordered ovarian cytochrome P450 activity and partly to increased LH stimulation.
- Peripheral insulin resistance occurs, with the resulting hyperinsulinaemia also promoting ovarian androgen production.

Clinical Features

- Amenorrhoea, oligomenorrhoea with long cycles, prolonged irregular bleeding at intervals less than 21 days or more than 35 days.
- Weight gain with increased abdominal fat. The BMI and the waist circumference should be measured.
- Hyperandrogenism may cause hirsutism, acne and acanthosis nigricans, but no virilism.
- Infertility and recurrent miscarriages.

Investigations

- Ultrasound scanning
- Laboratory tests
  - Elevated testosterone levels.
    - Free testosterone levels are elevated because sex hormone binding globulin (SHBG) levels are low. (Total testosterone divided by sex hormone binding globulin (SHBG) × 100 gives the free testosterone level.) Total

testosterone is normal or marginally elevated. If testosterone levels are greater than 5 nmol/L, a tumour is suspected.

– Elevated LH levels.
– Elevated LH:FSH ratio.
– Increased fasting insulin levels.
– Increased prolactin levels.
– Increased oestradiol and oestrone levels.

Ancillary Investigations

• Oral glucose tolerance test once a year in:
  – obese patients,
  – those with a family history of type 2 diabetes or a personal history of gestational diabetes mellitus,
  – elderly women over the age of 40 years.
• Lipid profile
• Transvaginal scan to assess endometrial thickness if there is prolonged amenorrhoea. Endometrial hyperplasia is less likely if the thickness is less than 7 mm.

Diagnosis

Two of the three following criteria are required to diagnose the condition—Rotterdam consensus criteria.

• Ultrasound evidence of polycystic ovaries:
  – 12 or more peripheral subcapsular follicles less than 10 cm in diameter.
  – Increased ovarian stroma and volume (greater than 10 cm^3).
• Oligo or anovulation.
• Clinical and/or biochemical evidence of hyperandrogenism.

An elevated luteinising hormone/follicle-stimulating hormone ratio is not regarded as a diagnostic criterion for PCOS owing to its inconsistency.

Differential Diagnosis

Thyroid dysfunction, congenital adrenal hyperplasia, hyperprolactinaemia, androgen-secreting tumours and Cushing's syndrome.

Associated Risks

• Cardiometabolic syndrome—hypertension, dyslipidaemia, visceral obesity, insulin resistance and hyperinsulinaemia, impaired glucose tolerance and type 2 diabetes.
• Endometrial carcinoma—anovulation causes high unopposed oestrogen levels, predisposing to development of endometrial carcinoma. There is no increased risk of breast and ovarian cancer.
• Pregnancy complications—gestational diabetes (OGTT should be done at 24–28 weeks), pre-eclampsia and preterm delivery.
• Non-alcoholic fatty liver.
• Depression.
• Obstructive sleep apnoea.

TREATMENT

There is no definite treatment for PCOS. Treatment should be directed at the symptoms which are most prominent and troublesome.

• Exercise and weight control
  – Lifestyle modification with changes in diet and exercise is the first line treatment, for obese patients with PCOS. Obesity increases insulin resistance. Weight loss will reduce the likelihood of developing type 2 diabetes later in life. Treatment with metformin for several months can cause a small reduction of body fat. Orlistat may also be used.
• Amenorrhoea/oligomenorrhoea/irregular bleeding
  – First line treatment of irregular bleeding is combined oral contraceptive pills for 3–6 months, if the patient does not need immediate fertility.
  – Cyclical norethisterone can be used for 1–3 cycles in infertile patients.
  – Progesterone can be used to cause withdrawal bleeding once in 3–4 months, to prevent endometrial hyperplasia in patients with amenorrhoea.
• Hirsutism
  – Cyproterone acetate, an anti-androgen, that competitively inhibits the andro-

gen receptors, is given in the form of DianetteM, (which consists of cyproterone 2 mg and 35 mcg of ethinyloestradiol) if the patient does not need immediate fertility.
- Cosmetic treatment.
• Infertility
- Weight reduction should be achieved first.
- Ovulation induction
  □ Clomiphene citrate 50–100 mg daily from 2nd–6th day of the menstrual cycle

□ Follicular tracking to detect a pre-ovulatory follicle.

□ Injection of hCG at mid-cycle when a pre-ovulatory follicle (1.8–2 cm) is present.

□ Letrozole 5 mg daily from 2nd–6th day of the menstrual cycle can be used in those not responding to clomiphene.

- Laparoscopy and diathermy cauterization of follicles is done in those not responding to medical treatment.

QUESTIONS

1. A 30-year-old athlete complains of amenorrhoea for 1 year. Her BMI is 20 kg/m². FSH and LH levels are within the low normal range. Clinical and ultrasound examinations are normal.

   What is the most likely cause?

   A. Anorexia nervosa.
   B. Depression.
   C. Excessive exercise.
   D. Premature menopause.
   E. Use of performance enhancing drugs.

2. A 30-year-old athlete complains of amenorrhoea for two years. Her BMI is 20 kg/m². Her FSH is 60 IU and LH level is 55 IU. Clinical and ultrasound examinations are normal.

   What is the most likely cause?

   A. Anorexia nervosa.
   B. Excessive exercise.
   C. Depression
   D. Premature menopause.
   E. Use of performance enhancing drugs.

3. A 25-year-old woman with one child complains of absence of menstruation for 3 years after her delivery. She had undergone an evacuation of retained placental tissue 10 days after her delivery. She had lactated for 1½ years. Her BMI is 20 kg/m². She has not used any

contraceptives. Urine hCG is negative. Abdominal ultrasound scan is normal.

What is the most likely diagnosis?

A. Asherman syndrome.
B. Cervical stenosis.
C. Hyperprolactinaemia.
D. Post-natal depression.
E. Sheehan's syndrome.

4. A 25-year-old unmarried woman complains of amenorrhoea for 3 months. She has noticed secretions from both breasts. Urine hCG is negative. Ultrasound examination is normal. FSH and LH levels are within the low normal range. She is not on any drugs. She denies any previous pregnancies. Her BMI is 24 kg/m².

   What is the first step in the management?

   A. Perform a CT scan of the brain.
   B. Perform serum prolactin levels.
   C. Test the visual fields.
   D. Treat with bromocriptine.
   E. Treat with OCP for three cycles.

5. A 25-year-old unmarried woman complains of amenorrhoea for 4 months. She has noticed secretions from both breasts. Urine hCG is negative. Ultrasound examination is normal. She is not on any drugs. She denies any previous pregnancies.

Her BMI is 24 kg/m^2. Serum prolactin is 1000 mIU/L.

What is the most appropriate next step in the management?

A. Preform a CT scan of the brain.

B. Perform a mammogram.

C. Perform an X-ray of the pituitary fossa.

D. Perform serum FSH and LH levels.

E. Test the visual fields.

6. A 25-year-old nulliparous woman complains of amenorrhoea for 4 months and secretions from both breasts. Urine hCG is negative. Ultrasound examination is normal. She is not on any drugs. She denies any previous pregnancies. Her BMI is 24 kg/m^2. Serum prolactin is 1000 mIU/L. CT scan reveals a pituitary microadenoma.

What is the most appropriate treatment?

A. Laser ablation of the tumour.

B. Radiotherapy.

C. Trans-sphenoidal resection of the microadenoma.

D. Treatment with bromocriptine.

E. Treatment with cabergoline.

7. A 30-year-old woman who has two children was on depot medroxyprogesterone acetate injections for two years. She has taken the last injection 4 months ago. She complains of amenorrhoea for two years. Her last child is two years of age. Her BMI is 25 kg/m^2. Urine hCG is negative. She wishes to conceive in the near future.

What is the best management option?

A. Await spontaneous onset of menstruation.

B. Commence ovulation induction with clomiphene citrate.

C. Give metformin for three months.

D. Give norethisterone for 7 days.

E. Give OCP for three cycles.

8. A 25-year-old woman complains of infrequent scanty periods and infertility. Her BMI is 30 kg/m^2.

Which of the following tests should be performed to confirm the diagnosis of polycystic ovarian syndrome?

A. Elevated LH:FSH ratio.

B. Increased fasting insulin levels.

C. Increased oestradiol levels.

D. Increased prolactin levels.

E. Ultrasound evidence of polycystic ovaries.

9. A 25-year-old unmarried woman complains of oligomenorrhoea and increased facial hair. Her BMI is 35 kg/m^2. Ultrasound scan of the ovaries reveal more than 12 subcapsular follicles and increased stroma.

What is the first step in the management?

A. Advise cosmetic treatment for hirsutism.

B. Advise lifestyle modification and weight reduction.

C. Commence ovulation induction with clomiphene citrate.

D. Treat with combined oral contraceptive pills for three months.

E. Treat with cyproterone acetate for 3 cycles.

10. A 35-year-old nulliparous woman who has been married for 3 years attends the infertility clinic. Her menstrual periods occur once in 45–60 days. She has increased facial hair. The BMI is 24 kg/m^2. Ultrasound scan reveals more than 12 subcapsular follicles in the ovaries with increased stroma.

What is the most appropriate first line treatment?

A. Commence ovulation induction with clomiphene citrate.

B. Perform laparoscopy and diathermy cauterisation of the ovaries.

C. Treat with combined oral contraceptive pills for three months.

D. Treat with metformin for three months.

E. Treat with monthly injections of GnRH analogues for three months.

11. **A 23-year-old unmarried woman complains of bleeding for three weeks, after a period of amenorrhoea of two months. She is worried about excess facial hair and acne. Her periods have been irregular for 2 years. Her BMI is 24 kg/m². Ultrasound scan reveals more than 12 subcapsular follicles in the ovaries with increased stroma. The endometrial thickness is 1 cm.**

What is the best treatment option?

A. Advice cosmetic treatment for hirsutism.

B. Commence ovulation induction with clomiphene citrate.

C. Give metformin for 3 months.

D. Treat with combined oral contraceptive pills for three months.

E. Treat with cyproterone acetate for 6 cycles.

12. **A 20-year-old unmarried girl presents with irregular periods and increased facial hair of 2 years duration. She gets only 3–4 periods per year. Bleeding is heavy and prolonged and lasts for 15–20 days. Her BMI is 30 kg/m². Plasma LH levels are elevated and the serum free testosterone is 3 nmol/L.**

What is the most likely diagnosis?

A. Adrenal tumour.

B. Arrhenoblastoma of the ovary.

C. Cushing's syndrome.

D. Polycystic ovarian syndrome.

E. Testicular feminization.

13. **A 30-year-old woman complains of infertility, irregular periods and increase of facial hair of 2 years duration. She gets only 3–4 scanty periods per year. Her BMI is 30 kg/m². Plasma LH levels are elevated. She wishes to conceive soon.**

What is the best treatment option?

A. Combined oral contraceptive pills.

B. Diathermy punctures of ovarian cysts.

C. Metformin and cyproterone acetate.

D. Pulsatile administration of GnRh.

E. Weight reduction and clomiphene citrate

14. **A 35-year-old woman with 3 children complains of amenorrhoea for 3 years. She is on depot medroxyprogesterone acetate injections for 3 years. Her BMI is 30 kg/m². Transvaginal ultrasound scan is normal. She does not wish to conceive again.**

What is the best treatment option?

A. Continue the DMPA injections and induce withdrawal bleeding with norethisterone once in 3 months.

B. Reassure and continue DMPA injections.

C. Stop the DMPA injections and commence on oral contraceptive pills.

D. Stop the DMPA injections and insert a copper containing intrauterine device.

E. Stop the DMPA injections and insert a levonorgestrel-releasing intrauterine device.

ANSWERS AND EXPLANATIONS

Q.1 (C)

This patient who is an athlete has no other abnormalities. FSH and LH levels are within the low normal range. Therefore, her amenorrhoea is most probably due to excessive exercise. FSH and LH levels should be high if she has gone into premature menopause. Although performance enhancing drugs can cause amenorrhoea, there is no mention regarding clinical features of using these drugs. The cause is unlikely to be anorexia nervosa because the BMI is normal.

Q. 2 (D)

This athlete has high FSH and LH levels. Therefore, her amenorrhoea is due to premature menopause. If it was due to excessive exercise, the FSH and LH levels should be in the low normal range.

Q. 3 (A)

This woman had undergone an evacuation of retained placental tissue 10 days after her delivery. Therefore, most likely cause of amenorrhoea is Asherman's syndrome, which is common after puerperal curettage. The presence of infection and low oestrogen levels during lactation favour adhesion formation. One of the characteristic symptoms of Sheehan's syndrome is failure of lactation. Since this woman had lactated for 1 ½ years the cause is unlikely to be Sheehan's syndrome. If there is cervical stenosis there should be a haematometron on the ultrasound scan. There is no mention regarding prolactin levels or symptoms of depression.

Q. 4 (B)

Q. 5 (A)

Explanation for questions 4 and 5

Hyperprolactinaemia due to a pituitary tumour should be considered if a nulliparous woman complains of secretions from the breasts with oligomenorrhoea or amenorrhoea. Therefore, the first step in the management is to perform serum prolactin levels. If the prolactin level is greater than 1000 mIU/L, a pituitary tumour should be suspected. The next step is to perform a CT scan of the brain. Visual fields also should be assessed. Pituitary macroadenomas require surgery. Microadenomas can be treated with cabergoline or bromocriptine.

Q. 6 (E)

The best treatment option for a pituitary microadenoma is cabergoline which is a dopamine agonist. The initial dose is 0.25 mg twice a week and may be increased up to 1 mg twice a week. It is preferred to bromocriptine because of the less frequent administration and lower incidence of side

effects. Bromocriptine is an alternative drug but daily or twice daily administration is necessary. The initial dose is 1.25–2.5 mg daily. The dose can be increased up to 2.5 mg twice daily which is the therapeutic dose. Surgery/laser ablation is recommended for macroadenomas of the pituitary.

Q. 7 (A)

Restoration of ovulation, menstruation and fertility takes a few months after cessation of depot medroxyprogesterone acetate injections. Therefore, the best option is to wait for spontaneous return of ovulation and menstruation. Induction of ovulation can be considered if she does not conceive after return of regular menstrual cycles. Treatment with OCP or norethisterone will result in withdrawal bleeding but will not restore ovulation.

Q. 8 (E)

A clinical diagnosis of PCOS can be made as she has 2 Rotterdam criteria required for diagnosis. She has infrequent scanty periods (clinical evidence of infrequent ovulation) and clinical evidence of hyperandrogenism. Diagnosis can be further confirmed if there is ultrasound evidence of polycystic ovaries with 12 or more peripheral subcapsular follicles less than $10 \ cm^3$ in diameter, increased ovarian stroma and volume (greater than $10 \ cm^3$). Elevated LH : FSH ratio increased fasting insulin levels, increased prolactin levels and increased oestradiol levels are biochemical changes which occur in PCOS, but are not regarded as diagnostic criteria.

Q. 9 (B)

Diagnosis of PCOS can be made as she has all three Rotterdam criteria required for diagnosis of this condition. The first line treatment for an obese patient with PCOS is lifestyle modification and weight reduction. Cyproterone is a better option than OCP to regularize her periods as it will improve the hirsutism as well.

Cosmetic treatment is also an option for hirsutism. Ovulation induction is not indicated as she is unmarried and does not desire fertility at present.

Q. 10 (A)

Diagnosis of PCOS can be made as she has all three Rotterdam criteria required for diagnosis of this condition. Since this patient is not obese and wishes to conceive as soon as possible, the first step in the management is to induce ovulation with clomiphene citrate and mid-cycle gonadotropin injections. Metformin is not indicated as she is not obese and OCP should not be given as she desires fertility as soon as possible. Diathermy cauterisation of the ovaries should be done only if ovulation induction fails after at least 3 cycles.

Q. 11 (E)

Diagnosis of PCOS can be made as she has all three Rotterdam criteria required for diagnosis of this condition. Treatment of PCOS should be directed towards the most prominent and the troublesome symptom. This patient has prolonged bleeding with infrequent irregular periods. She is worried about hirsutism and acne. Therefore, the best treatment option is to give cyproterone acetate for six cycles, to stop the continuous bleeding, to improve her hirsutism and acne and to regularise the periods. Cyproterone is a better option than OCP to regularize her periods as it will improve the hirsutism as well. However, cyproterone cannot be given if she desires immediate fertility. Metformin is not indicated as she is not obese. Ovulation induction is not indicated as she is unmarried and does not desire fertility at present. Cosmetic treatment will improve the hirsutism temporally, but will not settle the irregular menstruation.

Q. 12 (D)

The most likely diagnosis is PCOS because she has oligomenorrhoea and clinical and biochemical evidence of hyperandrogenism. Adrenal tumour and arrhenoblastoma of the ovary will cause a greater degree of virilism. Patients with Cushing's syndrome will have other signs such as moon face and truncal obesity. Testicular feminisation will cause primary amenorrhoea.

Q. 13 (E)

This woman is obese and has clinical features of PCOS. Since she is concerned about her infertility and wishes to conceive soon, the best treatment option is, life-style modification, weight reduction and ovulation induction with clomiphene citrate. Diathermy puncture of ovaries is done later if ovulation induction fails. Combined oral contraceptive pills and cyproterone will impair her fertility further.

Q. 14 (D)

This patient is having amenorrhoea due to prolonged use of DMPA injections for contraception. Use of OCP will induce monthly bleeding, but may result in post-pill amenorrhoea, once the treatment is stopped. OCP is best avoided after 35 years of age especially in obese women. Amenorrhoea will continue if a progesterone containing IUCD is inserted. Therefore, the best option is to insert a copper IUCD, which is an effective method of contraception without hormones. It is not necessary to induce withdrawal bleeding, as DMPA will cause endometrial atrophy and prevent endometrial hyperplasia.

REFERENCE

Gynaecology by Ten Teachers, 19th ed.

4

Postoperative Complications

STRUCTURES WHICH CAN BE DAMAGED AT HYSTERECTOMY

The ureter, bladder and bowel can be damaged at hysterectomy.

Pathway of the Ureter

Ureter crosses the pelvic brim at the bifurcation of the common iliac artery, runs on the lateral pelvic wall close to the ovarian fossa, enters the posterior leaf of the broad ligament, turns medially, and reaches the lateral edge of the uterosacral ligaments. It runs close to the vault of the vagina, crosses underneath the uterine artery and runs within 1.5 cm (or closer) to the cervix in the Mackenrodt's ligament. It runs forward and medially under the ligament, ascends anterior to the vagina for a short distance and reaches the base of the bladder. It opens into the bladder at the lateral angle of the vesical trigone.

INJURY TO THE URETER

Injury at Total Hysterectomy

The ureter can be injured at total hysterectomy (through an abdominal incision or through laparoscopy):

- while clamping the infundibulopelvic ligament at oophorectomy especially in the presence of endometriosis or malignancy,
- in the ovarian fossa during resection of ovaries or ovarian remnants,
- while suturing the vault of the vagina because the ureter runs close to the vault of the vagina before entering the trigone of the bladder,
- while dividing the uterosacral ligaments especially in the presence of endometriosis,
- while clamping the Mackenrodt's ligament and the uterine artery to remove the cervix (the commonest site).

Ureter cannot be damaged while pushing the bladder down to expose the cervix, as it does not run on the anterior leaf of the broad ligament.

Injury to the ureter is less likely to occur at subtotal hysterectomy as the cervical stump is clamped at a higher level.

The left ureter is at a greater risk of damage as it lies closer to the uterus.

Injury to the Ureter at Vaginal Hysterectomy

Ureter is pulled downwards when traction is applied on the cervix, which is one of the first steps of vaginal hysterectomy. This is more prominent in the case of a third/fourth degree prolapse.

Therefore, the ureter can be damaged while ligating the cardinal ligament and the uterine artery.

However, ureteric damage can be prevented if the bladder is pushed up, above the fundus of the uterus and is reflected laterally, as the ureter will move away from the surgical field.

Symptoms

A direct injury to the ureter will result in leaking of urine soon after the surgery. Ligation of the ureter, ischaemia due to impairment of the blood supply or passage of a stitch through the ureter, will cause necrotic damage and leaking of urine 4–5 days later.

Symptoms of Undetected Ureteric Injuries in the Postoperative Period

- Fever with chills.
- Haematuria or oliguria.
- Flank pain.
- Abdominal distension with peritonitis/ileus.
- Abscess formation/sepsis.
- Urinary leakage (vaginally or via the abdominal wound).
- Ureteral stricture, hydronephrosis, renal damage/ renal failure.
- It should be noted that typical symptoms may be absent in up to 50% of women.

Treatment

The surgical procedures used to treat ureteral injury are removal of a ligature, ureteral stenting, ureteral resection and ureteroureterostomy, transureteroureterostomy and ureteroneocystostomy.

INJURY TO THE BLADDER

The bladder can be damaged at total abdominal hysterectomy while:
- entering into the peritoneal cavity,
- dissecting the utero vesical peritoneum,
- pushing the bladder down to expose the cervix,
- removing the cervix,
- suturing the anterior flap of the vaginal vault.

The bladder can be damaged at vaginal hysterectomy while:
- pushing the bladder/cystocele up to expose the fundus,

- entering the peritoneal cavity from the anterior aspect.
- A stitch can go through the full thickness of the bladder while repairing the cystocele.

Treatment

- Most extraperitoneal bladder injuries heal with catheter drainage for 10–14 days.
- Those which fail to heal need surgical repair.
- If the injury is detected at surgery immediate repair gives good results.

Occurrence of Postoperative Fistulae

- Leaking of urine through the vagina soon after surgery with the catheter *in situ* is due to cutting the ureter or due to a large cut in the bladder.
- Leaking of urine through the vagina soon after removing the catheter is due to a cut in the bladder.
- Leaking of urine 4–5 days after surgery is due to ligation, passage of a suture or ischaemic necrosis of the bladder or the ureter.

OTHER URINARY COMPLICATIONS

Oliguria

- An intake output chart should be maintained for at least 48 hours after major surgery.
- Oliguria occurs due to inadequate fluid replacement and should be detected and treated early.
- Treatment is with intravenous fluid replacement.

Urinary Retention

- The woman should be encouraged to pass urine within 6 hours after surgery.

- Retention is usually caused by pain.
- The first step in the treatment is pain relief, followed by catheterisation if the patient fails to pass urine.
- If retention recurs after catheterisation, an indwelling catheter should be inserted for 48 hours.
- If not detected and treated, retention with overflow can occur. This condition can mimic a fistula.
- Urine should be sent for full report, culture and antibiotic sensitivity test.

Urinary Tract Infection

- Occurs after 48 hours.
- It is a cause of postoperative fever.
- The first step is to send the urine for full report, culture and antibiotic sensitivity test.
- A broad spectrum antibiotic such as ciprofloxacin, norfloxacin or cephalosporin is commenced, till the results of the antibiotic sensitivity test is available.

POSTOPERATIVE FEVER

If fever occurs within,
- – 0–2 days—fibrin fever due to tissue damage.
- – 2–3 days—urinary tract infection, respiratory tract infection, peritonitis.
- – 3–5 days—wound infection, pelvic abscess (swinging fever), deep vein thrombosis, urinary tract infection, respiratory tract infection, cannula site infection.
- It is treated with broad spectrum antibiotics after identifying the infecting organism. An abscess should be drained.

Occurrence of Bowel Injury at Abdominal Hysterectomy

- The small bowel can be damaged while opening into the peritoneal cavity.
- The large bowel and the rectum can be damaged while removing the cervix and

suturing the posterior flap of the vaginal vault.

Occurrence of Bowel Injury at Vaginal Hysterectomy

- The small bowel can be damaged while opening into the peritoneal cavity from the posterior aspect (pouch of Douglas) and while repairing the enterocele.
- The rectum can be damaged while repairing the rectocele.

ABDOMINAL DISTENSION/VOMITING

- Paralytic ileus
  - – Occurs 24–48 hours after surgery due to excessive handling of the bowel.
  - – Causes vomiting and abdominal distension with sluggish bowel sounds.
  - – Is treated with intravenous fluids and nasogastric suction.
- Peritonitis
  - – Occurs 48–72 hours after surgery due to infection.
  - – Fever and vomiting may be present.
  - – Abdomen will be distended with tenderness and guarding. Bowel sounds will be sluggish.
  - – Treated with intravenous fluid, nasogastric suction and intravenous broad spectrum antibiotics.
- Bowel injury
  - – Manifests 24–48 hours after surgery.
  - – Fever will occur due to infection. Abdominal pain and vomiting will occur. The patient will be ill.
  - – Abdomen will be distended with tenderness and guarding.
  - – USS will show free fluid in the peritoneal cavity.
  - – X-ray erect abdomen will show air under the diaphragm.
  - – Surgery should be performed immediately.

POSTOPERATIVE HAEMORRHAGE

Reactionary Bleeding

- Occurs in the first 24 hours.
- It is mild and is due to capillary bleeding.
- Treated with a pressure dressing.

Slip Ligature

- Occurs in the first 24 hours.
- It causes severe haemorrhage due to slipping of the uterine or ovarian pedicle.
- The patient may complain of sweating, shoulder tip pain and chest pain.
- There will be signs of haemodynamic compromise such as, low blood pressure, tachycardia and pallor.
- There will be signs of blood in the peritoneal cavity such as, abdominal distension, tenderness, guarding and flank dullness.
- There may be restlessness, dyspnoea and low urine output.
- Treated with resuscitation and immediate laparotomy.

Secondary Haemorrhage

- Occurs 5–14 days after surgery.
- Caused due to infection followed by sloughing of the infected tissue, exposing the underlying blood vessels.
- It is a rare complication which occurs mostly after vaginal procedures. It could occur after abdominal hysterectomy due to infection at the vaginal vault.
- May be preceded by fever and vaginal discharge.
- Resuscitation and blood transfusion is required in severe cases.
- Bleeding is arrested by inserting a tight vaginal pack. It is not possible to cauterize or ligate the blood vessels, as the infected tissues are very friable and handling can aggravate the bleeding.
- Intravenous broad spectrum antibiotics should be given.

WOUND INFECTION, HAEMATOMA, ABSCESS AND DEHISCENCE

- Occur from 4 to 10 days.
- Cause pain and discharge from the wound and fever.
- If a haematoma or an abscess is found, it should be drained by opening the wound under local anaesthesia.
- Pus should be cultured and an intravenous broad spectrum antibiotic should be commenced till the report is available.
- Wound should be cleaned and dressed daily with hypertonic saline. Secondary suturing should be done when the wound is clean.
- Wound dehiscence commences within 24-48 hours, but manifests in 4–7 days when the dressing is removed.
- Can be suspected by the presence of a serous discharge from the wound.
- Wound dehiscence is treated with analgesics, intravenous broad spectrum antibiotics and immediate suturing under general anaesthesia. All the layers of the abdominal wall are sutured together using non-absorbable suture material.

Pelvic Abscess

- Causes abdominal pain, high swinging fever, abdominal tenderness and guarding. Signs of peritonitis will be present if there is free pus in the peritoneal cavity.
- Diagnosis is confirmed by ultrasound scanning, which will show a localised abscess, or the presence of thick free fluid in the peritoneal cavity.
- Intravenous broad spectrum antibiotics should be commenced and changed after the results of the ABST.
- A localised abscess can be drained under ultrasound guidance. Laparotomy is needed if the abscess is inaccessible, or if the pus is too thick for aspiration, or if there is free pus in the peritoneal cavity. Pus should be sent for culture and antibiotic sensitivity test.

1. A woman who underwent an uncomplicated abdominal hysterectomy develops abdominal distension and starts to leak urine through the vagina within the first 24 hours, while she is on catheter drainage.

   Which one of the following injuries could most likely have happened during the operation?

   A. Cutting the ureter at the infundibulopelvic ligament.
   B. Cutting the ureter while removing the cervix.
   C. Injuring the bladder while dissecting the utero vesical peritoneum.
   D. Ligation of the ureter at the cardinal ligament.
   E. Ligation of the ureter while suturing the vault of the vagina.

2. A woman who was in labour for 12 hours undergoes a mid-cavity forceps delivery. She starts to leak urine through the vagina 7 days after delivery. Post-voidal scan of the bladder does not show any residual urine.

   Which of the following is the most likely cause of her symptoms?

   A. Injury to the bladder during the forceps delivery.
   B. Injury to the ureter during the forceps delivery.
   C. Necrosis of an area of the bladder due to prolonged pressure by the foetal head.
   D. Pressure on the ureter during the forceps delivery.
   E. Retention with overflow.

3. A woman starts to leak urine through the vagina 7 days after vaginal hysterectomy and repair. Post-voidal scan of the bladder does not show any residual urine.

Which of the following is the most likely cause of her symptoms?

A. Detrusor instability.
B. Injury to the bladder during the surgery.
C. Injury to the ureter during the operation.
D. Passage of a suture through the full thickness of the bladder during the cystocele repair.
E. Retention with overflow.

4. A woman develops fever 24 hours after an uncomplicated abdominal hysterectomy.
   Which one of the following is the most likely cause?
   A. Fibrin fever due to tissue damage.
   B. Peritonitis.
   C. Upper respiratory tract infection.
   D. Wound dehiscence.
   E. Wound infection.

5. A woman develops a temperature of 38°C 4 days after an uncomplicated abdominal hysterectomy.
   Which one of the following is the most likely cause?
   A. Fibrin fever due to tissue damage.
   B. Paralytic ileus.
   C. Peritonitis.
   D. Wound dehiscence.
   E. Wound infection.

6. A woman develops a temperature of 38°C 48 hours after an uncomplicated abdominal hysterectomy.
   Which one of the following is the most likely cause?
   A. Fibrin fever due to tissue damage.
   B. Pelvic abscess.
   C. Upper respiratory tract infection.
   D. Wound dehiscence.
   E. Wound infection.

7. A woman develops swinging fever rising up to 39°C 5 days after an uncomplicated hysterectomy.

   Which one of the following is the most likely cause?

   A. Paralytic ileus.

   B. Peritonitis.

   C. Pelvic abscess.

   D. Upper respiratory tract infection.

   E. Wound dehiscence.

8. A woman develops profuse vaginal bleeding 7 days after vaginal hysterectomy. This was preceded by fever and offensive vaginal discharge for three days.

   What is the most likely cause?

   A. Disseminated intravascular coagulation.

   B. Disturbance of granulation tissue due to straining at stools.

   C. Rupture of a pelvic abscess.

   D. Secondary haemorrhage.

   E. Slipped ligature.

9. A woman develops profuse vaginal bleeding 7 days after vaginal hysterectomy. This was preceded by fever and offensive vaginal discharge for three days.

   What is the best treatment option?

   A. Application of a figure of eight suture to the raw area.

   B. Emergency laparotomy to find the bleeding vessel.

   C. Ligation of the bleeding vessels through a vaginal approach.

   D. Tight packing of the vagina.

   E. Transfusion of platelets and fresh frozen plasma.

10. Which one of the following is the commonest site of ureteric damage during an uncomplicated total hysterectomy and bilateral salpingo-oophorectomy?

   A. While applying the first uterine clamp.

   B. While dissecting the utero vesical peritoneum.

   C. While ligating the infundibulopelvic ligament.

   D. While removing the cervix.

   E. While suturing the vault of the vagina.

11. A woman is restless 4 hours after hysterectomy. She complains of abdominal pain, chest pain and difficulty in breathing. There is no vaginal bleeding. The catheter is draining clear urine. On examination she is pale. Her blood pressure is 80/60 mmHg and the pulse rate is 130 bpm. The abdomen is tender with guarding and flank dullness is present.

   What is the most appropriate management?

   A. Inform the Senior Register.

   B. Keep under observation if the patient's condition improves after blood transfusion.

   C. Perform a laparotomy as soon as possible after resuscitation.

   D. Perform an ultrasound scan to confirm intraperitoneal bleeding.

   E. Relieve pain by giving an intramuscular injection of 75 mg of pethidine.

11a. A woman is restless 5 hours after hysterectomy. She complains of severe abdominal pain. There is no vaginal bleeding. The catheter is draining clear urine. Her blood pressure is 120/80 mmHg, the pulse rate is 90 bpm and the respiratory rate is 22. The abdomen is soft and tender. She has not been given any drugs after the operation.

   What is the most appropriate initial management?

A. Give 100% oxygen by face mask.

B. Give 1000 ml of 10% dextrose.

C. Give an intramuscular injection of 75 mg of pethidine.

D. Perform a laparotomy as soon as possible.

E. Perform an ultrasound scan to exclude intraperitoneal bleeding.

12. **A woman who had undergone an abdominal hysterectomy 5 days ago complains of watery blood stained discharge from the abdominal wound. When the dressing is opened the wound is found to have given way completely.**

What is the most appropriate treatment?

A. Apply through and through sutures immediately after giving intravenous antibiotics.

B. Suture after giving intravenous antibiotics for 48 hours.

C. Suture after the infection subsides completely.

D. Admit to the ICU for treatment of shock.

E. Suture each layer separately, immediately.

13. **A woman develops swinging fever rising up to 39°C and a pulse rate of 130 beats per minute, with abdominal pain, diarrhoea and vomiting, 5 days after an uncomplicated hysterectomy. An ultrasound scan reveals a localised pelvic abscess measuring 6 × 8 cm.**

What is the first step in the management?

A. Drain the abscess after treating with antibiotics for 24 hours.

B. Drain the abscess through a laparotomy and culture the pus.

C. Drain the abscess under ultrasound guidance and culture the pus.

D. Perform daily ultrasound scans.

E. Send a blood culture and commence intravenous broad spectrum antibiotics.

13a **A woman develops swinging fever rising up to 39°C and a pulse rate of 130 beats per minute, with abdominal pain, diarrhoea and vomiting, 5 days after an uncomplicated hysterectomy. An ultrasound scan reveals a localised pelvic abscess measuring 6 × 8 cm. Intravenous broad spectrum antibiotics are commenced.**

What is the next step in the management?

A. Drain the abscess through a laparotomy and culture the pus.

B. Drain the abscess through laparoscopy and culture the pus.

C. Drain the abscess under ultrasound guidance and culture the pus.

D. Perform daily ultrasound scans after commencing antibiotics.

E. Treat with broad spectrum antibiotics for two weeks.

14. **A woman develops throbbing pain in the wound 4 days after an uncomplicated abdominal hysterectomy. Her temperature is 37.8°C and the general condition is satisfactory. On examination a tender red swelling is found at one end of the wound.**

What is the next step in the management?

A. Drain the wound after treating with antibiotics for 24 hours.

B. Drain the wound immediately and culture the pus.

C. Dress the wound with hypertonic saline.

D. Perform a blood culture and commence intravenous broad spectrum antibiotics.

E. Perform an ultrasound scan to exclude pelvic infection.

15. **A woman has not passed urine for 8 hours after an abdominal hysterectomy. She complains of abdominal pain. On examination the bladder is distended. There are no other abnormalities.**

What is the first step in the management?

A. Catheterize once.

B. Encourage to pass urine.

C. Give analgesics to relieve pain.

D. Improve hydration.

E. Insert an indwelling catheter.

16. **A woman complains of urinary incontinence 4 days after an abdominal hysterectomy. She gives a history of passing urine several times a day. On examination the bladder is distended. Post-voidal ultrasound scan reveals a large volume of residual urine. There are no other abnormalities.**

What is the first step in the management?

A. Catheterize once.

B. Encourage to pass urine.

C. Give analgesics to relieve pain.

D. Insert an indwelling catheter for 48 hours.

E. Perform a cystoscopy to detect a vesicovaginal fistula.

ANSWERS AND EXPLANATIONS

Q. 1 (B)

Ligation of the ureter will not result in leaking of urine till sloughing occurs after about 5 days. Bladder injury will not cause leaking of urine till the catheter is removed, unless if the injury is very large. Only a direct injury to the ureter can cause leaking of urine soon after surgery with the catheter *in situ*. Ureteric ligation and injuries commonly occur while ligating and cutting the cardinal ligaments to remove the cervix, because the ureter is closest to the uterus at this point. It is rare to damage the ureter at the infundibulopelvic ligament, as the ureter runs close to the lateral pelvic wall at this level.

Q. 2 (C)

If there is retention with overflow post-voidal scan of the bladder will show residual urine. The ureter cannot be injured during forceps delivery. If the bladder is injured during the forceps delivery, the woman should start leaking urine soon after the procedure. Therefore, the fistula is caused by necrosis of an area of the bladder due to prolonged pressure by the foetal head. This part could slough off in about 5 days causing a fistula.

Q. 3 (D)

If there is retention with overflow post-voidal scan of the bladder will have residual urine. If the bladder is injured during the surgery, she will start leaking urine as soon as the catheter is removed. If the ureter is injured during surgery, the urinary leak will commence soon after surgery. Passage of a suture through the full thickness of the bladder during the anterior repair and sloughing of the damaged tissue, can cause a fistula about 5–7 days after surgery. Detrusor instability will cause urgency and not true incontinence.

Q. 4 (A)

Q. 5 (E)

Q. 6 (C)

Q. 7(C)

Explanation for questions 4, 5, 6 and 7

Fibrin fever due to tissue damage will occur within the first 24-48 hours after surgery. Upper respiratory tract infection can develop in 48 hours. Peritonitis will cause fever in 48–72 hours. Paralytic ileus will manifest in 24-48 hours and may not cause fever. Wound infection will cause fever in 4–5 days. A pelvic abscess will occur in 5–7 days and will result in high swinging fever. Wound dehiscence will manifest in 5–7 days and may or may not cause fever.

Q. 8 (D)

Q. 9 (D)

Explanation for questions 8 and 9

Bleeding due to a slipped ligature will occur within the first 24 hours. Disturbance of granulation tissue will cause mild bleeding. There is no reason for her to develop disseminated intravascular coagulation (DIC) and there is no clinical evidence to suggest DIC. Rupture of a pelvic abscess will cause discharge of pus. This patient developed bleeding 7 days after the surgery and it was preceded by fever and offensive vaginal discharge. Therefore, the most likely cause is secondary haemorrhage, due to infection and sloughing of the infected tissue, exposing the underlying blood vessels. In secondary haemorrhage after vaginal hysterectomy, the raw bleeding area is in the vagina. The treatment is to apply pressure on the bleeding area by inserting a tight vaginal pack. It is not possible to ligate or cauterize the individual bleeding vessels, or to apply a figure of eight suture as the tissues are very friable. Laparotomy is not indicated as the bleeding is from the vagina.

Q. 10 (D)

The ureter is closest to the uterus when it crosses under the uterine artery and runs within 1.5 cm of the cervix in the Mackenrodt's ligament, which has to be clamped to remove the cervix. Therefore, the ureter is most likely to be damaged when removing the cervix. The ureter runs on the lateral pelvic wall close to the ovarian fossa and can be damaged if the infundibulopelvic ligament is cut very laterally, as in the case of an ovarian malignancy. A stitch can pass through the ureter when suturing the vault of the vagina. The ureter is less likely to be damaged when placing the first uterine clamp, as at this level it runs lateral to the uterus, in the posterior leaf of the broad ligament. The ureter cannot be damaged when dissecting the utero-vesicle peritoneum, as it runs in the posterior leaf of the broad ligament.

Q. 11 (C)

This patient has signs of intra-peritoneal bleeding with haemodynamic compromise, most probably due to a slip ligature. The most appropriate treatment is to perform a laparotomy and ligate the slipped pedicle as soon as possible. Senior staff members should be informed immediately. Blood transfusion is necessary, but surgery should not be postponed if the patient's condition improves after giving blood. Intra-peritoneal bleeding is an emergency situation and should be diagnosed clinically. Ultrasound scanning can be used to confirm the diagnosis, but is not essential. Pethidine should not be given till her haemodynamic condition is stable.

Q. 11a (C)

The commonest cause of restlessness in the immediate postoperative period is pain. Others are hypoxia, haemorrhage and urinary retention. Haemorrhage and hypoxia can be excluded in this woman because the vital parameters are within the normal range. There is no urinary retention as the catheter is draining clear urine. Therefore, the restlessness is most probably due to pain and the first step in the management is to relieve pain.

Q. 12 (A)

Wound dehiscence occurs early in the postoperative period, but manifests in about 4–5 days when the dressing is removed. However, wound dehiscence should be suspected, if the dressing appears to be wet with a serous pinkish discharge. Once dehiscence is diagnosed antibiotics should be commenced, pain should be relieved and the wound should be sutured immediately, under general or spinal anaesthesia. All the layers of the abdominal wall are sutured together using non-absorbable suture material.

Q. 13 (E) and Q. 13a (C)

A diagnosis of severe sepsis is made because this patient has high fever, tachycardia, vomiting and diarrhoea. The first step in the management is to perform a blood culture to isolate the organism. Next intravenous broad spectrum antibiotics are commenced and may be changed later, when the results of the antibiotic sensitivity tests are available.

The pelvic abscess should be drained after commencing broad spectrum anti-biotics, because the focus of sepsis has to be removed to improve the patient's condition. The pus should be sent for culture and ABST. Drainage is first attempted by aspiration under ultrasound guidance because the abscess is localised. Laparotomy is done only if aspiration fails. Aspiration may fail due to inaccessibility of the abscess, or due to increased thickness of the pus. Laparoscopy is not used to drain an abscess in the presence of severe sepsis. Ultrasound scans are done daily after aspiration of the abscess to exclude recurrence.

Q. 14 (B)

This woman has developed an abscess in the wound. Since she is not septic it is not necessary to perform a blood culture. The first step in the management is to open the wound under local anaesthesia and drain the abscess and culture the pus. Next intravenous broad spectrum antibiotics are commenced and may be changed later when the results of the antibiotic sensitivity tests are available. Wound is dressed daily with hypertonic saline. Secondary suturing is done when the wound is clean and free of pus. An ultrasound scan may be performed to exclude pelvic infection.

Q. 15 (C)

The commonest cause of urinary retention in the immediate postoperative period is pain. Therefore, the first step is to give analgesics to relieve pain. She should be encouraged to pass urine. If these measures fail, she should be catheterized. If retention recurs after catheterisation, an indwelling catheter should be inserted and kept *in situ* for 48 hours. Hydration is not essential as the bladder is distended indicating formation of urine.

Q. 16 (D)

When a woman develops urinary incontinence 4 days after surgery, a fistula caused by ligating the ureter, or passage of a stitch through the full thickness of the bladder and sloughing of the ischaemic tissue, should be first considered. Therefore, the first step is to perform a scan to determine filling of the bladder. In this case the bladder was distended and the post-voidal scan showed a large amount of residual urine. Therefore, the urinary leak is due to undiagnosed urinary retention, resulting in bladder atony with retention and overflow. The presence of urinary retention may be missed in cases like this, as the patient continued to pass urine. The best treatment option is catheter drainage for 48–72 hours, to keep the bladder empty and to regain muscle tone. Subsequently the catheter is clamped for 2–3 hours and released several times, before it is ultimately removed.

5

Contraception

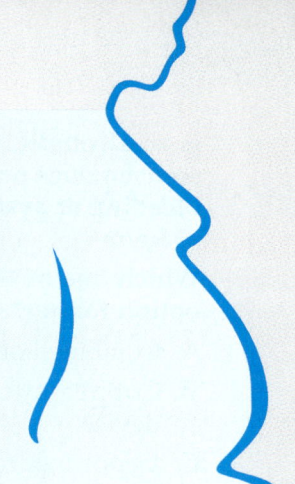

Please refer the articles given below for:

- indications and contraindications for the use of different methods of contraception,

- guidelines for selection of a suitable method of contraception,

- Medical eligibility criteria for contraceptive use.

A summary of the theory is not included in this chapter as a summary of all the necessary details are found in these articles.

- UK Medical Eligibility Criteria for Contraceptive Use. Faculty of Sexual and Reproductive Healthcare, Royal College of Obstetricians and Gynaecologists.
- Medical eligibility criteria for contraceptive use 5th ed., 2015. World Health Organization.
- U.S. Selected Practice Recommendations for Contraceptive Use, 2013. Adapted from the World Health Organization Selected Practice Recommendations for Contraceptive Use, 2nd ed.

QUESTIONS

1. A 25-year-old woman with tight mitral stenosis, who has delivered her first baby 6 weeks ago, seeks contraceptive advice.

   Which one of the following methods would be the best option for her?

   A. Combined oral contraceptive pills.

   B. Condoms.

   C. Copper bearing intrauterine contraceptive device.

   D. Levonorgestrel-releasing intrauterine system.

   E. Progestogen only subdermal implant.

2. A 35-year-old woman with tight mitral stenosis and pulmonary hypertension, who has just delivered her second baby, seeks contraceptive advice.

   Which one of the following methods would be the best option for her?

   A. Condoms.

   B. Interval sterilization by laparoscopy in 6 weeks.

   C. Interval sterilization by minilaparotomy in 6 weeks.

   D. Postpartum sterilization.

   E. Progestogen only subdermal implant.

3. A 26-year-old woman with three children seeks family planning advice. Her last child is 6 weeks of age. She is having marital problems because her husband

is an alcoholic. Her periods are regular and she does not have heavy menstrual bleeding or dysmenorrhoea. Her BMI is 35 kg/m².

Which one of the following is the best option for her?

A. Combined oral contraceptive pills.

B. Copper intrauterine contraceptive device.

C. Depot medroxyprogesterone acetate injections.

D. Permanent sterilization.

E. Levonorgestrel-releasing intrauterine device.

4. A 19-year-old nulliparous girl consults you for family planning advice two months prior to her wedding. She has been educated up to grade 5. She has regular periods with primary dysmenorrhoea. Her BMI is 23 kg/m².

What is the best of the following options?

A. Combined oral contraceptive pills.

B. Condoms.

C. Copper intrauterine contraceptive device.

D. Progestogen only subdermal implant.

E. Progestogen only pills.

5. A 41-year-old woman who has just delivered her second baby seeks contraceptive advice. There is no history of dysmenorrhoea, heavy menstrual bleeding or medical problems.

Which one of the following methods would be the best option?

A. Combined oral contraceptive pills.

B. Condoms.

C. Copper bearing intrauterine device.

D. Depot medroxyprogesterone acetate injections.

E. Permanent sterilization.

6. A 32-year-old mother of 2 children who has diabetes mellitus seeks contraceptive advice. Her diabetic condition is not

well controlled. There is no history of dysmenorrhoea or heavy menstrual bleeding. Her BMI is 30 kg/m².

What is the best option for her?

A. Combined oral contraceptive pills.

B. Copper intrauterine device.

C. Depot medroxyprogesterone acetate injections.

D. Levonorgestrel releasing intrauterine device.

E. Permanent sterilization.

7. A 30-year-old mother of one child who developed deep vein thrombosis 4 days after delivery by caesarean section seeks contraceptive advice. Her child is 6 months old and her thrombosis was successfully treated. Her BMI is 35 kg/m².

What is the best option for her?

A. Combined oral contraceptive pills.

B. Copper intrauterine device.

C. Depot medroxyprogesterone acetate injections.

D. Levonorgestrel-releasing intrauterine device.

E. Progestogen only subdermal implant.

8. A 33-year-old woman who has undergone chemotherapy for carcinoma of the breast seeks contraceptive advice. She has one child who is 5 years of age.

What is the best option for her?

A. Combined oral contraceptive pills.

B. Copper intrauterine device.

C. Depot medroxyprogesterone acetate injections.

D. Levonorgestrel-releasing intrauterine device.

E. Progestogen only subdermal implant.

9. A 35-year-old woman with two children who has undergone chemotherapy for carcinoma of the breast seeks contraceptive advice.

What is the best option for her?

A. Combined oral contraceptive pills.

B. Copper intrauterine device.

C. Levonorgestrel-releasing intrauterine device.

D. Permanent sterilisation.

E. Progestogen only subdermal implant.

10. A 25-year-old woman with one child seeks contraceptive advice. She gives a history of clear mucoid vaginal discharge. The cervix appears inflamed on speculum examination. Her husband is working abroad and comes home once in 2 months.

Which one of the following methods would be the best option for her?

A. Combined oral contraceptive pills.

B. Condoms.

C. Copper intrauterine device.

D. Depot medroxyprogesterone acetate injections.

E. Progestogen only subdermal implant.

11. A 36-year-old woman with two children seeks contraceptive advice. Her last child is 1 year of age. She has had bleeding once in two to three weeks with excessive flow during the past four months. Clinical examination and ultrasound scanning did not reveal any abnormalities.

Which one of the following methods would be the best option?

A. Combined oral contraceptive pills.

B. Copper intrauterine device.

C. Depot medroxyprogesterone acetate injections.

D. Levonorgestrel-releasing intrauterine device.

E. Progestogen only subdermal implant.

12. A 32-year-old woman, who has one child, seeks contraceptive advice for a period of two years. She has primary dysmenorrhoea and frequent irregular menstrual bleeding. No abnormalities are detected on examination or ultrasound scanning.

What is the best contraceptive method for her?

A. Combined oral contraceptive pills.

B. Depot medroxyprogesterone acetate injections.

C. Levonorgestrel-releasing intrauterine device.

D. Progestogen only pills.

E. Progestogen only subdermal implant.

13. A 25-year-old woman who has one child seeks contraceptive advice. She has had viral hepatitis one month ago. Liver enzymes are slightly elevated but the coagulation profile is normal.

What is the best contraceptive method for her?

A. Combined oral contraceptive pills.

B. Copper intrauterine device.

C. Depot medroxyprogesterone acetate injections.

D. Progestogen implant.

E. Progestogen only pills.

14. A woman who had a caesarean section for the delivery of her second baby 25 days ago seeks contraceptive advice. Her BMI is 30 kg/m². She has a past history of heavy menstrual bleeding.

Which of the following is the best method for her?

A. Combined oral contraceptive pills.

B. Condoms.

C. Copper intrauterine device.

D. Depot medroxyprogesterone acetate injections.

E. Progestogen implant.

15. A woman who has delivered her first child 6 weeks ago seeks contraceptive advice. She suffers from frequent attacks of migraine with aura.

Which of the following is the best method for her?

A. Combined oral contraceptive pills.

B. Copper intrauterine device.

C. Depot medroxyprogesterone acetate injections.

D. Levonorgestrel-releasing intrauterine system.

E. Progestogen implant.

16. A 25-year-old woman whose second pregnancy ended in a hydatidiform mole six weeks ago seeks contraceptive advice. Serum β-hCG levels are still elevated.

Which of the following is the best method for her?

A. Combined oral contraceptive pills.

B. Condoms.

C. Copper intrauterine device.

D. Levonorgestrel-releasing intrauterine system.

E. Progestogen implant.

17. A woman whose second pregnancy ended in a hydatidiform mole 50 days ago seeks contraceptive advice. Serum β-hCG levels are normal. She does not wish to conceive soon.

Which of the following is the best method for her?

A. Condoms.

B. Copper intrauterine device.

C. Oral contraceptive pills.

D. Progestogen implant.

E. Progestogen only pills.

18. A 39-year-old woman, who had eclampsia at 34 weeks during her second pregnancy, seeks contraceptive advice 3 months after the delivery. Her blood pressure is 160/110 mmHg. Her baby is healthy.

What is the best method of contraception for her?

A. Condoms.

B. Copper intrauterine device.

C. Levonorgestrel-releasing intrauterine system.

D. Permanent sterilization.

E. Progestogen only subdermal implant.

19. A 32-year-old mother of two children seeks contraceptive advice. Her first child is 4 years old and the second child is 2 years old. She has developed hypertension 2 years ago. Her blood pressure is 160/110 mm Hg. She has heavy menstrual bleeding for 1 year.

What is the best method of contraception for her?

A. Combined oral contraceptive pills.

B. Copper intrauterine device.

C. Depot medroxyprogesterone acetate injections.

D. Levonorgestrel-releasing intrauterine system.

E. Permanent sterilization.

20. A woman who is taking combined oral contraceptive pills misses 2 consecutive pills. There are 10 pills remaining in the packet.

Which of the following is the safest option?

A. Take both pills immediately, continue the packet and use condoms for 7 days.

B. Take the most recent missed pill immediately, continue the packet and use condoms for 7 days.

C. Take the most recent missed pill immediately, start a new packet immediately and use condoms for 7 days.

D. Take the most recent missed pill immediately, use condoms for 7 days, continue the packet and commence the next packet after a 7 days gap.

E. Take the most recent missed pill immediately, use condoms for 7 days, continue the packet and commence the next packet without a 7 days gap.

21. A 39-year-old woman with 3 children who is using condoms requests emergency contraception 4 days after an act of unprotected intercourse.

Which of the following is the best option?

A. 1.5 mg of levonorgestrel.

B. 100 mcg of ethinyloestradiol and 0.5 mg of levonorgestrel.

C. Copper intrauterine device.

D. DMPA injection.

E. Progestogen only subdermal implant.

22. **A 25-year-old nulliparous woman who is using condoms requests emergency contraception 12 hours after an act of unprotected intercourse.**

    Which of the following is the best option?

    A. 1.5 mg of levonorgestrel.

    B. 100 mcg of ethinyloestradiol and 0.5 mg of levonorgestrel.

    C. Copper intrauterine device.

    D. DMPA injection.

    E. Progestogen only subdermal implant.

23. **A 30-year-old woman who has delivered her first child 6 weeks ago seeks contraceptive advice. She has a submucous fibroid and had heavy frequent bleeding before she became pregnant. She wishes to have a myomectomy before her next pregnancy. She is exclusively breast-feeding her baby.**

    What is the best method for her?

    A. Combined oral contraceptive pills.

    B. Condoms.

    C. Copper bearing intrauterine device.

    D. Levonorgestrel-releasing intrauterine system.

    E. Progestogen implant.

24. **Woman who had an IUCD inserted 1 year ago attends the clinic for a routine check-up. On vaginal examination the threads of the IUCD are not found. Attempts to retrieve threads using a cervical cytology brush failed.**

    What is the next step in the management?

A. Dilate the cervix and explore the uterus under general anaesthesia.

B. Perform a CT scan.

C. Perform a transvaginal ultrasound scan

D. Perform an X-ray of the pelvis after inserting another IUCD

E. Perform an X-ray of the pelvis.

25. **Woman who had an IUCD inserted 1 year ago attends the clinic for a routine check-up. On vaginal examination the threads of the IUCD are not found. The IUCD is found to be in the correct position within the uterus on ultrasound scanning.**

    What is the best management option?

    A. Leave the IUCD in the uterus.

    B. Remove the IUCD after dilating the cervix under general anaesthesia.

    C. Remove the IUCD after dilating the cervix with vaginal misoprostol.

    D. Remove the IUCD using a long artery forceps.

    E. Remove the IUCD using a thread retriever.

26. **Woman who had a copper IUCD inserted 10 years ago wishes to remove it. On vaginal examination the threads of the IUCD are not found. The IUCD is found to be in the correct position within the uterus on ultrasound scanning.**

    What is the best management option?

    A. Leave the IUCD in the uterus anticipating spontaneous expulsion.

    B. Remove the IUCD after dilating the cervix under general anaesthesia.

    C. Remove the IUCD after dilating the cervix with vaginal misoprostol.

    D. Remove the IUCD using a long artery forceps.

    E. Remove the IUCD using a thread retriever.

ANSWERS AND EXPLANATIONS

Q. 1 (E)

Even though barrier methods do not carry any cardiac risks they are best avoided, because their efficacy is low and are user dependant and are hence not reliable. Combined hormonal contraceptive pills should be avoided because of the risk of thrombosis and fluid retention. These risks can be minimised by using progestogen-only preparations. Levonorgestrel containing intrauterine device is an option because it is very efficient. Its contraceptive efficacy is superior to that of sterilisation. It causes oligomenorrhoea/ amenorrhoea, thereby preventing anaemia. In contrast copper devices can cause menorrhagia and dysmenorrhoea. The risk of endocarditis is less with LNGIUS than with copper devices. The cardiovascular risk of the IUCD is confined to the time of insertion, in particular to instrumentation of the cervix, which can cause a vasovagal reaction in up to 5% of women. A progestogen implant is effective, safe and is not user dependant. It does not carry a risk of subacute bacterial endocarditis or any other cardiac risk and is therefore the best choice. Patients with heart disease should be advised to complete their family early and the ideal interval between two children is 2 years.

Q. 2 (C)

Sterilisation is the best option as she is 39 years old, has 2 children and has pulmonary hypertension. Insufflation of the peritoneal cavity with carbon dioxide, the head down tilt and positive pressure ventilation, required during laparoscopic sterilization will reduce the cardiac output. There is also a risk of air embolism. The safest and the best method is sterilization by minilaparotomy under spinal anaesthesia. Interval sterilization is safer than post-partum sterilization, as the cardiovascular changes of pregnancy will return to normal by that time. A progestogen implant can be inserted if she refuses sterilization.

Q. 3 (B)

Even though this woman has three children, she is young and might seek a divorce, as she is having marital problems. Therefore, permanent sterilisation should be avoided and a long-term reversible contraceptive method should be considered. Progestogen contained in contraceptives, especially DMPA can cause weight gain and is not suitable as her BMI is 35. Moreover, she might not visit the clinic regularly once in 3 months for the injection. OCP is not suitable as it is user dependant and she may not take the pills regularly without missing. Also OCP carries an increased risk of venous thromboembolism in obese women. The best option is a copper intrauterine contraceptive device, as this needs changing only once in 10 years and needs only a single act of motivation. Also she has no history of menorrhagia or dysmenorrhoea. A levonorgestrel-releasing intrauterine device is also a suitable option, but it is expensive and is not freely available in hospital practice.

Q. 4 (D)

Condoms and oral contraceptives are user dependant and the woman may not be motivated to use them regularly. Irregular use with subsequent failure is more likely in this woman, as she is young and not well educated. There may be technical difficulties to insert an IUCD and poor acceptance in a nulliparous woman. Therefore, a progestogen implant is the best option, as it needs a single act of motivation once in 3–5 years depending on the brand. Jadelle is effective for 5 years. The effects are reversed when the device is removed. Jadelle implants are a set of two flexible cylindrical implants, each containing

75 mg of levonorgestrel. The progestogen implants release a small amount of etonogestrel 25–70 mcg daily. Jadelle may interact with phenytoin, phenobarbital and carbamazepine. Progestogen only pills have a high failure rate.

Q. 5 (E)

Since this woman is 41 years of age and has two children the best option would be permanent sterilization. If she refuses sterilization, a copper intrauterine device is a good option, as she has no abnormal menstrual bleeding and it provides effective contraception for 10 years, by which time she may reach menopause. OCP is not recommended for women over 35 years, because of the increased risk of cardiovascular disease and thrombosis. These effects are more in obese patients and diabetics. Condoms are user dependant and are not regarded as a foolproof method.

Q. 6 (B)

All hormonal contraceptives are best avoided in women with diabetes (especially if poorly controlled or if complications are present). Reversible long-term contraception is a better option than permanent sterilisation as she is 32 years of age and has 2 children. A copper bearing intrauterine device is the best option for this patient. However, a levonorgestrel-releasing intrauterine device can be used in a diabetic patient, if a copper IUCD cannot be inserted due to abnormal menstrual bleeding.

Q. 7 (B)

Hormonal contraceptives are best avoided in women with a history of venous thrombosis. Therefore, a copper intrauterine device would be the best option, as it has no effect on the venous thrombosis and provides long-term reversible contraception. A LNGIUS can be inserted if there are contraindications

for a copper intrauterine device, such as dysmenorrhoea or heavy menstrual bleeding.

Q. 8 (B)

This patient needs reversible long-term contraception as she has only one child. Copper intrauterine device is the best option, as all hormonal contraceptives are contraindicated in women with breast carcinoma. If the woman has heavy menstrual bleeding, LNGIUS is the only option.

Q. 9 (D)

Pregnancy can cause recurrence and spread of carcinoma of the breast. Since this woman has two children permanent sterilisation is the best option. If she refuses sterilisation a copper intrauterine device is the next best option, as it would provide long-term reversible contraception, without hormonal influence.

Q. 10 (B)

Since she seems to be having chlamydial infection and the husband is coming home once in 2 months, condoms would be the best option. Condoms will also protect her from acquiring other sexually transmitted infections. However, condoms and OCP are user dependant and will fail if not taken regularly. An intrauterine contraceptive device should not be inserted in the presence of chlamydial/pelvic infection. However, if this woman cannot be relied upon to use condoms, a progestogen implant would be an option, as it provides continuous contraception for 3–5 years, depending on the brand.

Q. 11 (D)

A levonorgestrel containing intrauterine system is the best option for this patient, as it will provide long-term effective contraception, while providing a cure for her abnormal menstrual bleeding. Sometimes it can cause irregular spotting, but the effects will be reversed, as soon as the device is removed. A progestogen implant will have the same effects and is a suitable option. OCP will also provide relief from her menstrual irregularity, but is a temporary method, which is user dependant and is not recommended for women over the age of 35 years. Copper containing IUCD can aggravate her menstrual problem. The disadvantages of DMPA are the need of an injection once in three months, the occurrence of prolonged amenorrhoea and irregular spotting, which can persist for some time after stopping treatment.

Q. 12 (A)

OCP would be the best option because if taken regularly it would provide short-term contraception and relief from dysmenorrhoea and irregular menstrual bleeding. If she cannot be motivated to take OCP regularly, LNGIUS or a progestogen implant are suitable options, but these are more suitable for long-term reversible contraception. Also they can cause amenorrhoea or irregular spotting, but the effects are reversed once the device is removed. The disadvantages of DMPA are requirement of an injection once in three months and the occurrence of prolonged anovulation, with amenorrhoea or irregular spotting, which can persist after stopping treatment. Fertility may not return for some time after stopping treatment.

Q. 13 (B)

Since all hormones are metabolised in the liver hormonal contraceptives should be avoided in those with impaired liver function. A copper bearing IUCD is the best option in this patient. However, heavy menstrual bleeding can occur if the coagulation profile is abnormal.

Q. 14 (E)

This woman has a risk of venous thrombo-embolism, as she is obese and is in the puerperal period after a caesarean section. Therefore, OCP is best avoided. DMPA causes weight gain and is not suitable as she is already obese. Copper intrauterine device can cause heavy menstrual bleeding. Condoms are user dependant and therefore the failure rate is high. The best option is a progestogen implant as it can be kept for 3–5 years and will reduce the menstrual blood loss, or cause amenorrhoea. The amount of progesterone released daily is very small and will not cause weight gain.

Q. 15 (B)

Since she has migraine with aura all hormonal contraceptives are contraindicated. Therefore, a copper intrauterine device is the best option. A LNGIUS may be used if there are contraindications for the use of a copper containing intrauterine device.

Q. 16 (B)

Women with GTD should use a barrier method of contraception, until hCG levels revert to normal. Therefore, condoms would be the best option. However, condoms are user dependant and the patient should be motivated to use them at every act of intercourse. Intrauterine contraceptive devices should not be used until hCG levels are normal, to reduce the risk of perforating the soft uterus.

Q. 17 (D)

Once the serum B hCG levels are normal any method of contraception can be used. Since she does not wish to conceive soon, a progestogen implant would be the best option. However, they can cause irregular bleeding. Care is required to insert a copper intrauterine device into the soft uterus and it can cause irregular and heavy menstrual bleeding.

Q.18 (D)

This patient probably has essential hypertension as her blood pressure remains elevated after the puerperium. She is 39 years of age and has reached the end of the safe age for reproduction and has two children. She had a life threatening complication during the second pregnancy and most probably has pre-existing severe hypertension. Therefore, permanent sterilisation would be the best option. However, the woman should be appropriately counselled about the permanency of sterilization and the availability of highly effective, long-acting, reversible methods of contraception. If the woman refuses sterilization a copper containing intrauterine device is a good option, as it can be retained for 10 years. LNGIUS is not contraindicated in the presence of hypertension and is an option especially if the patient has a history of abnormal menstrual bleeding. Progestogen implants release a small amount of etonogestrel 25–70 mcg daily and is not contraindicated for patients with hypertension. Condoms are not recommended as they are user dependant and have a high failure rate.

Q. 19 (D)

Permanent sterilization is not recommended as she is 32 years of age and has 2 very young children and there are highly effective, long-acting, reversible methods of contraception. Since this patient has severe hypertension and needs suitable long-term contraception, till her hypertension is under control, LNGIUS is the best option. It would provide effective contraception for five years and would cure her menstrual problem. Copper containing intrauterine device is contraindicated, as it would aggravate her menstrual problem. OCP and DMPA are best avoided as she has severe hypertension.

Q. 20 (D)

The correct procedure to follow when a woman misses one or two pills is to take the most recent missed pill immediately, use condoms for 7 days and continue the packet. If 7 or more pills are remaining in the packet, finish the remaining tablets and start the next packet after a 7 days gap. If there are fewer than 7 pills remaining in the packet, finish the remaining tablets and start the next packet the next day without a 7 days gap.

Q. 21 (C)

Insertion of an intrauterine device or oral levonorgestrel 1.5 mg is effective for emergency contraception, if taken within 5 days of unprotected intercourse. However, emergency contraception should be taken as soon as possible after unprotected intercourse. Copper intrauterine device is the best method for this patient, as she is 39 years of age and long-term contraception would be a better option than condoms for her. Also an intrauterine device is effective to prevent implantation, if inserted within 5 days, before the embryo reaches the uterus.

Q. 22 (A)

The best option for this woman is 1.5 mg of levonorgestrel taken as a single tablet or two 0.75 mg tablets taken 12 hours apart. This is effective up to 5 days of intercourse, but is not effective after the implantation process commences. It is not known to harm the foetus if a woman inadvertently takes the pill after she becomes pregnant. It will not cause abortion. A copper intra-uterine device is not a suitable option as she is a nulliparous woman. However, she should be advised to use OCP or a subdermal implant, which are more reliable methods than condoms.

Q. 23 (E)

OCP should be avoided by women who are breastfeeding babies less than 6 months of age. Also OCP and condoms are user dependant and are not suitable for this woman, as she needs long-term reversible contraception, till the myomectomy is performed. An intrauterine device cannot be inserted, as the endometrial cavity may be distorted by the fibroid. A progestogen implant is the best option, as it will provide effective long-term contraception, while reducing the menstrual blood loss. Also progestogens do not reduce milk production or cause increased growth of the fibroid.

Q. 24 (C), Q. 25 (A) and Q. 26 (E)

If the threads of an IUCD are not felt the next step in the management is to detect whether it has been expelled or whether it is in the uterus or in the peritoneal cavity.

The first step is to perform a transvaginal ultrasound scan.

If the IUCD is found in the correct position in the uterus, the best option is to leave it *in situ*. However, if the time has expired or the patient wishes to remove it the best option is to use a thread retriever or a long artery forceps. Dilatation of the cervix with misoprostol is tried if these methods fail. Dilatation under general anaesthesia is rarely necessary.

6

Benign and Malignant Ovarian Tumours

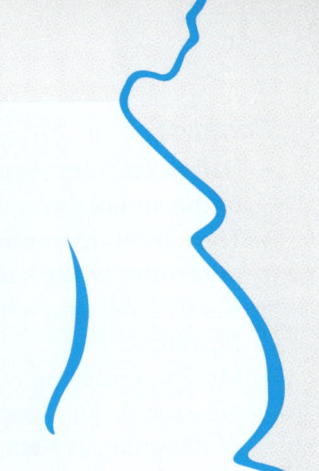

PHYSIOLOGICAL CYSTS

- May occur in premenopausal women. They are most common in young women. They do not occur after menopause.
- Most are asymptomatic, incidental findings at pelvic examination or ultrasound scan.
- They are smaller than 7.5 cm, thin walled and unilocular.
- They are an occasional complication of ovulation induction, when they are commonly multiple.
- They are follicular or luteal cysts.

BENIGN NEOPLASMS

Benign Germ Cell Tumours

- Mature cystic teratoma
- Mature solid teratoma
- Rise from totipotential germ cells.
- They contain elements of all three germ layers.

Dermoid Cyst (Mature Cystic Teratoma)

- The benign dermoid cyst is the only benign germ cell tumour that is common.
- It is bilateral in about 11% of cases.
- It is an unilocular cyst less than 15 cm in diameter, in which ectodermal structures are predominant.
- Thus it is often lined with epithelium like the epidermis and contains skin appendages, teeth, sebaceous material, hair and nervous tissue.
- Endodermal derivatives include thyroid, bronchus and intestine, and the mesoderm may be represented by bone, cartilage and smooth muscle.

Benign Epithelial Tumours

- Serous cystadenoma
- Mucinous cystadenoma
- Endometrioid cystadenoma
- Clear cell (mesonephroid) tumour
- Brenner tumour
- Arise from the ovarian surface epithelium.
- They are therefore mesothelial in nature, deriving from the coelomic epithelium overlying the embryonic gonadal ridge, from which develop müllerian and wolffian structures.

Benign Sex Cord Stromal Cell Tumours

- Theca cell tumours
- Fibroma
- Sertoli-Leydig cell tumours and granulosa cell tumours are low grade malignant tumours.
- They occur at any age, from pre-puberty to post-menopause
- Many secrete hormones and present with the results of inappropriate hormone effects.

Fibroma

- Is derived from stromal cells and are similar to thecomas.
- They are hard, mobile and lobulated with a glistening white surface.
- Ascites occurs with many of the larger fibromas.
- Meig's syndrome where ascites and pleural effusion occur in association with a fibroma of the ovary is seen in only 1% of cases.

Presentation of Benign Ovarian Cysts

- Abdominal discomfort.
- Abdominal swelling.
- In most patients ovarian cysts do not cause symptoms and are detected at routine examination, or routine scanning.
- Pain will occur if there is torsion, infection, haemorrhage or rupture.
- Pressure effects will occur only when the cyst is very large.
- As a rule ovarian tumours do not cause hormonal effects and menstrual disturbances. Granulosa cell tumours and theca cell tumours produce oestrogen and arrhenoblastomas produce androgen.
- Symptoms suggestive of endometriosis should be specifically considered.
- Sometimes the woman may notice a lump.

Diagnosis

- On abdominal examination a cystic mass will be felt to one side of the midline.
- The surface will be smooth, margins well-defined, non-tender, mobile in both directions and it is possible to reach below the mass.
- Presence of free fluid in the peritoneal cavity should be excluded by percussion.
- On bimanual examination a cystic mass can be felt separate from the uterus.
- The diagnosis is confirmed by transvaginal and transabdominal USS.
- Transvaginal scanning in combination with colour flow mapping and 3D imaging may improve sensitivity, particularly in complex cases.
- CA-125 levels should be done to exclude malignancy, especially in postmenopausal women.
- A serum CA-125 assay is not essential in all premenopausal women, when an ultrasonographic diagnosis of a simple ovarian cyst has been made.
- Lactate dehydrogenase (LDH), alpha-fetoprotein and hCG levels should be estimated in all women less than 40 years of age with a complex ovarian mass, to exclude the occurrence of germ cell tumours.

The Value of CA-125 in Screening for Malignant Ovarian Tumours

- CA-125 is primarily a marker only for epithelial ovarian carcinoma.
- However, false positive results are common.
- CA-125 is raised in many benign conditions including fibroids, endometriosis, adenomyosis and pelvic infections. Therefore, a raised level should be interpreted with caution.
- Consequently if serum CA-125 is raised, but less than 200 units/ml, further investigations are required to exclude the common differential diagnoses.
- It may be helpful to carry out serial monitoring of CA-125 levels, as rapidly rising levels are more likely to be due to malignancy.

Calculation of the RMI

Calculation of the RMI is based on:
- serum CA-125 (CA-125);
- menopausal status (M);
- ultrasound score (U).

RMI = U × M × CA-125 (units/ml).

The ultrasound score is calculated by awarding 1 point each for:
- multilocular cysts,
- solid areas,
- metastases,

 - ascites,
 - bilateral lesions,

U = 0 (for an ultrasound score of 0), U = 1 (for an ultrasound score of 1), U = 3 (for an ultrasound score of 2–5).

The following score is calculated for menopausal status.

1 = premenopausal and 3 = postmenopausal.

Women who have had no period for more than one year or women over the age of 50 who have had a hysterectomy are regarded as postmenopausal.

Serum CA-125 can vary between zero and hundreds or even thousands of units/ml.

RMI	Risk of malignancy
Low <25	<3%
Moderate 25–250	20%
High >250	75%

Specific ultrasound features derived from the IOTA study can be used without CA-125 values to predict malignancy with high sensitivity, specificity and likelihood ratios.

B Rules for Benign Cysts

- Unilocular cysts.
- Presence of solid components where the largest solid component is less than 7 mm.
- Presence of acoustic shadowing.
- No blood flow.
- Smooth multilocular tumour with the largest diameter less than 100 mm.

M Rules for Malignant Cysts

- Irregular solid tumour.
- Ascites.
- Presence of at least 4 papillary structures.
- Irregular, multilocular, solid tumour with the largest diameter greater than 100 mm.
- Very strong blood flow.

(From RCOG Guideline No. 62)

Management in Premenopausal Women

- Simple ovarian cysts less than 50 mm diameter do not require follow-up. They are most probably physiological and usually disappear within 3 menstrual cycles.

- Simple ovarian cysts of 50–70 mm in diameter are followed up with yearly ultrasound scans. If persistent should be considered for either further imaging (MRI) or surgical intervention.
- Larger simple cysts and cysts that persist or increase in size are unlikely to be functional and may need surgery.

Surgical Procedures

- The laparoscopic approach is preferred for benign ovarian cysts, due to lower post-operative morbidity and shorter recovery time.
- Laparotomy is done for large masses, or for those with solid components, such as large dermoid cysts.
- Aspiration of ovarian cysts under ultrasound guidance or laparoscopically, is associated with a high rate of recurrence and is not recommended.
- The standard surgical procedure is cystectomy. The ovary is reconstructed and preserved.
- Oophorectomy is done in twisted gangrenous cysts, or if malignancy is suspected.
- If malignancy is suspected, the RMI score or specific ultrasound features should be used, to guide the management.

Malignancy is suspected at surgery if:
 - the tumour has breached the capsule,
 - there are large blood vessels on the surface,
 - the tumour has solid areas,
 - there are bilateral tumours,
 - there is ascites,
 - there are peritoneal or omental deposits.

- If malignancy is suspected oophorectomy is done, with a full thickness biopsy of the other ovary.
- If malignancy is confirmed by the presence of tumour deposits or free fluid, total abdominal hysterectomy, bilateral salpingo-oophorectomy and omentectomy is done, if the woman has completed her family.

Use of Laparoscopy in the Management of Ovarian Cysts

- Laparoscopy may be used for ovarian cystectomy in patients at low risk for ovarian cancer.
- The following ultrasound features should be present. The mass should be confined to one ovary and smaller than 10 cm. It must have a thin intact capsule and no solid parts, and there should be no ascites or any other evidence of spread.
- The serum CA-125 level must be normal (<35 U/mL).

OVARIAN CYSTS IN POSTMENOPAUSAL WOMEN

Require assessment with:
- transvaginal scan,
- CA-125,
- Calculation of RMI.

Low Risk Patients—Less than 3% Risk of Cancer

- Are managed in a gynaecology unit.
- Conservative management is carried for simple cysts smaller than 5 cm in diameter, with a CA-125 level of less than 30 units/ml. Ultrasound scans and serum CA-125 measurement should be done, every four months, for one year.
- Laparoscopic oophorectomy is recommended, if the cyst does not fit the above criteria, or if the woman requests surgery.

Moderate Risk Patients—Approximately 20% Risk of Cancer

- Are preferably managed in a cancer unit.
- Laparoscopic oophorectomy, with removal of the ovary intact in a bag without rupture of the cyst into the peritoneal cavity, is acceptable in selected cases.
- If malignancy is suspected at laparoscopy, a laparotomy should be done and a full staging procedure should be undertaken.

High Risk Patients—Greater than 75% Risk of Cancer

- Management in a cancer centre.
- Laparotomy should be done.

MALIGNANT OVARIAN TUMOURS

Diagnosis

Symptoms

Early ovarian cancer may not cause any symptoms or may cause only minimal, nonspecific symptoms. An abdominal mass may be felt at a later stage.

Most patients do not have symptoms till the disease is advanced. Hence the disease is diagnosed at a later stage.

Symptoms Are Non-specific and Vague

- Bloating, abdominal distension or discomfort.
- Pressure effects on the bladder and rectum.
- Indigestion and acid reflux.
- Shortness of breath.
- Tiredness.
- Weight loss.
- Early satiety.
- Menstrual disturbances occur only with hormone secreting tumours.

Signs

- A solid or cystic and solid abdomino-pelvic mass is felt. The mobility may be restricted due to adhesions and infiltration of the surrounding structures.
- Presence of free fluid.

Investigations

- CA-125
- Lactate dehydrogenase (LDH), alpha feto-protein and hCG should be measured in all women under 40 years of age, with a complex ovarian mass, to exclude germ cell tumours.
- Ultrasound scanning.

- Calculation of the RMI.
- CT scan of the abdomen and pelvis to determine the extent of the disease.

FIGO Staging of Ovarian Tumours

T1	I	Tumour limited to the ovaries (one or both)
T1a	IA	Tumour limited to one ovary; capsule intact, no tumour on ovarian surface; no malignant cells in ascites or peritoneal washings.
T1b	IB	Tumour limited to both ovaries; capsules intact, no tumour on ovarian surface; no malignant cells in ascites or peritoneal washings.
T1c	IC	Tumour limited to one or both ovaries with any of the following: capsule ruptured, tumour on ovarian surface, malignant cells in ascites or peritoneal washings.
T2	II	Tumour involves one or both ovaries with pelvic extension.
T2a	IIA	Extension and/or implants on the uterus and/or tube(s); no malignant cells in ascites or peritoneal washings.
T2b	IIB	Extension to and/or implants in other pelvic tissues; no malignant cells in ascites or peritoneal washings.
T2c	IIC	Pelvic extension and/or implants (T2a or T2b) with malignant cells in ascites or peritoneal washings.
T3	III	Tumour involves one or both ovaries with microscopically confirmed peritoneal metastasis outside the pelvis.
T3a	IIIA	Microscopic peritoneal metastasis beyond the pelvis (no macroscopic tumour).
T3b	IIIB	Macroscopic peritoneal metastasis beyond the pelvis 2 cm or less in greatest dimension.

Contd.

IIIC	Macroscopic peritoneal metastasis beyond the pelvis >2 cm in greatest dimension and/or regional lymph node metastasis.
IV	Distant metastases.

TREATMENT

- Laparotomy is performed for all ovarian cysts where there is a suspicion of malignancy, as indicated by a high risk of malignancy index.
- Surgery is the first line treatment for ovarian cancer.
- The aim of surgery is to confirm the diagnosis, stage the extent of disease, and resect all visible tumour deposits.
- The surgery is done through a wide midline incision.
- Tumour staging should be performed. This includes :
  - cytology of ascetic fluid or peritoneal washings.
  - multiple peritoneal biopsies.
  - biopsies from adhesions and suspicious areas.
  - omentectomy.
  - bilateral pelvic and para-aortic lymph node sampling.
  - diaphragmatic scraping or biopsy for cytology studies.
- The standard surgical procedure is total abdominal hysterectomy, bilateral salpingo-oophorectomy and infracolic omentectomy.
- If macroscopic disease is visible outside the ovary, all visible tumour deposits should be excised. This may involve radical surgery, including bowel resection and excision of peritoneal implants.
- Debulking surgery is done if complete removal of the tumour is not possible, as the prognosis depends mainly on the volume of residual disease at the completion of surgery.

Prognosis of advanced ovarian cancer can be classified in three groups based on the volume of residual disease at the completion of surgery:

- Good risk—Microscopic disease outside the pelvis (stage IIIa) or macroscopic disease less than 2 cm outside the pelvis (stage IIIb)
- Intermediate risk—Macroscopic disease less than 2 cm outside the pelvis after surgery
- Poor risk—Macroscopic disease more than 2 cm after surgery or disease outside the peritoneal cavity.

Interval Debulking

- Is performed if adequate debulking was not possible, at the time of initial surgery,
- is carried out after three cycles of postoperative chemotherapy. Optimal debulking would be possible in approximately 60% of patients.

Treatment of Stage IA Disease in Patients who wish for Future Fertility

- If there is no macroscopic disease outside the ovary, perform unilateral salpingo-oophorectomy and careful surgical staging of the disease.
- Remove the ovary and ovarian tumor intact and perform infracolic omentectomy.
- A full thickness biopsy of the other ovary should be done.

Chemotherapy

- Only patients with stage IA grade 1 and stage IB grade 1, serous, mucinous, endometrioid and Brenner tumours can be treated with surgery alone.
- Clear-cell carcinomas have a worse prognosis in stage I and should be considered for chemotherapy at all stages.
- These patients should be treated with a taxane/platinum (cisplatin or carboplatin) combination for 3 to 6 cycles.

- Radiotherapy is not routinely used in the treatment of ovarian cancer.
- Hormone replacement therapy should be used with caution and is contraindicated in those with endometrioid tumours.

TUMOUR MARKERS

CA-125

- About 90% of ovarian cancers are coelomic epithelial carcinomas and contain a coelomic epithelium related glycoprotein, designated cancer antigen 125.
- CA-125 is elevated in most serous, endometrioid, and clear cell ovarian carcinomas. Mucinous tumours express this antigen less frequently.
- CA-125 may also be raised in a number of other gynecologic (e.g. endometrium, fallopian tube) and non-gynecologic (e.g. pancreas, breast, colon, lung) cancers.
- However, elevation is most marked (>1500 units/ml) in epithelial ovarian cancer.
- False-positive results are common and may occur with endometriosis, adenomyosis, pelvic inflammatory disease, menstruation, uterine fibroids, or benign cysts.

β-hCG

- Beta-hCG is elevated in patients with choriocarcinoma, embryonal carcinomas, polyembryomas, mixed cell tumours, and, less commonly in dysgerminomas.
- β-hCG levels are assessed to determine the response to treatment and recurrence of gestational trophoblastic neoplasia.

Alpha-fetoprotein

- AFP is elevated in endodermal sinus tumour. AFP is also elevated in ovarian embryonal cell carcinoma, immature teratomas, and polyembryomas
- AFP and beta-hCG levels are used to assess the response to treatment and recurrence and play an important role in the

management of nonseminomatous germ cell tumours.

- Elevation of AFP and beta-hCG levels are less marked in early stage I disease and are hence of no value in screening for these tumours.

Inhibin

- Elevation of inhibin in a postmenopausal woman or a premenopausal woman presenting with amenorrhea and infertility may indicate the presence of a granulosa cell tumour. However, it is not a specific test.

- Inhibin levels are used for tumour surveillance after treatment, to assess for residual or recurrent disease.

Oestradiol

- Oestradiol is elevated in granulosa cell tumours. It is not a sensitive marker for these tumours.

Müllerian Inhibiting Substance (MIS)

MIS is undetectable in postmenopausal women. Therefore, an elevated MIS value is highly specific for ovarian granulosa cell tumours.

QUESTIONS

1. **A 30-year-old woman with one child complains of abdominal discomfort. Ultrasound scan reveals a smooth walled tumour 8 cm × 8 cm, with a hyperechoeic nodule 6 mm in diameter with multiple thin echogenic bands, arising from the right ovary. The capsule is intact. Internal blood flow is not seen on the colour Doppler scan. The left ovary and the other organs are normal. There is no free fluid.**

   What is the most appropriate treatment?
   A. Hysterectomy and bilateral salpingo-oophorectomy.
   B. Keep under observation for 3 months if CA-125 is within normal limits.
   C. Ovarian cystectomy.
   D. Ultrasound guided aspiration and cytology of the fluid.
   E. Right salpingo-oophorectomy.

2. **A 49-year-old woman complains of abdominal discomfort and lower abdominal distension. Ultrasound scan reveals a smooth 8 × 6 cm tumour, with a solid nodule 9 mm in diameter, rising from the left ovary. The capsule is intact. The right ovary is normal. There is no free fluid. The other organs are normal.**

   What is the most appropriate treatment?

   A. Hysterectomy and bilateral salpingo-oophorectomy.
   B. Hysterectomy and unilateral salpingo-oophorectomy.
   C. Ovarian cystectomy.
   D. Ultrasound guided aspiration and cytological examination of the fluid.
   E. Unilateral salpingo-oophorectomy.

3. **A 45-year-old woman complains of abdominal discomfort and lower abdominal distension. Ultrasound scan reveals a 14 × 16 cm multilocular cyst, with thin septa, arising from the right ovary. There are no solid areas. There is no evidence of free fluid or metastatic lesions. Internal blood flow is not seen on the colour Doppler scan.**

   What is the most appropriate management?

   A. Hysterectomy and bilateral salpingo-oophorectomy.
   B. Laparoscopy and right salpingo-oophorectomy.
   C. Laparotomy and ovarian cystectomy.
   D. Laparotomy and right salpingo-oophorectomy.
   E. Ultrasound guided aspiration and cytological examination of the fluid.

3a. **A 30-year-old woman with 1 child complains of abdominal discomfort and lower abdominal distension. Ultrasound scan reveals a 14 × 16 cm multilocular cyst, with thin septa, arising from the right ovary. There are no solid areas. There is no evidence of free fluid or metastatic lesions. Internal blood flow is not seen on the colour Doppler scan.**

What is the most appropriate management?

A. Hysterectomy and bilateral salpingo-oophorectomy.

B. Laparoscopy and right salpingo-oophorectomy.

C. Laparotomy and ovarian cystectomy.

D. Laparotomy and right salpingo-oophorectomy.

E. Ultrasound guided aspiration and cytological examination of the fluid.

4. **A 25-year-old unmarried woman presents with a history of abdominal discomfort and distension. Ultrasound scan reveals a 12 cm × 14 cm solid mass arising from the right ovary, a smaller solid mass in the left ovary and free fluid. At laparotomy a solid ovarian tumour is found in the right ovary and a smaller solid tumour in the left ovary. Tumour deposits are found in the pouch of Douglas. There is free fluid in the peritoneal cavity. CA-125 is 1500 IU/ml and alpha fetoprotein is undetectable.**

What is the most appropriate management?

A. Three cycles of chemotherapy followed by total abdominal hysterectomy and bilateral salpingo-oophorectomy.

B. Total abdominal hysterectomy and bilateral salpingo-oophorectomy with infracolic omentectomy followed by chemotherapy.

C. Total abdominal hysterectomy and bilateral salpingo-oophorectomy with infracolic omentectomy followed by radiotherapy.

D. Total abdominal hysterectomy and bilateral salpingo-oophorectomy and chemotherapy.

E. Unilateral salpingo-oophorectomy, infracolic omentectomy and full thickness biopsy of the other ovary.

5. **A 25-year-old nulliparous woman presents with a history of abdominal discomfort. Ultrasound scan reveals a 8 cm × 9 cm solid mass arising from the right ovary. The left ovary is normal and there is no free fluid. Serum alpha-fetoprotein levels are elevated. At surgery a solid ovarian tumour with an intact capsule is found. It is confined to the right ovary. There is no free fluid or metastases.**

What is the most appropriate treatment?

A. Laparoscopy, unilateral salpingo-oophorectomy, infracolic omentectomy and full thickness biopsy of the other ovary.

B. Laparotomy, unilateral salpingo-oophorectomy, infracolic omentectomy and full thickness biopsy of the other ovary.

C. Six cycles of chemotherapy followed by cystectomy.

D. Six cycles of chemotherapy followed by oophorectomy.

E. Total abdominal hysterectomy and bilateral salpingo-oophorectomy with infracolic omentectomy.

6. **A 22-year-old woman complains of sudden onset of lower abdominal pain and vomiting. A tender mass is found in the right iliac fossa. Ultrasound scan reveals an ovarian tumour 8 × 7 cm with a 6 mm hyperechoeic nodule (Rokitansky nodule) and multiple thin echogenic bands rising from the right ovary. The capsule of the tumour is intact and there is no internal blood flow on the colour Doppler scan. The other ovary is normal. There is no free fluid. CA-125 level is normal.**

What is the most appropriate treatment?

A. Aspirate the ovarian cyst under ultrasonic guidance.

B. Perform a laparotomy and ovarian cystectomy.

C. Perform a laparotomy and unilateral oophorectomy.

D. Perform laparoscopic ovarian cystectomy.

E. Review in the clinic if the pain subsides.

7. A 30-year-old woman, who has been infertile for 2 years, complains of dysmenorrhoea and dyspareunia. She has menstruation once in 20–25 days. Ultrasound scan reveals an ovarian mass 8 cm × 7 cm with echogenic fluid.

What is the most appropriate method of management?

A. Continuous treatment with oral contraceptive pills for 6 months followed by surgical excision.

B. Laparoscopic unilateral salpingo-oophorectomy.

C. Laparoscopic cystectomy followed by treatment with oral danazol for 6 months.

D. Laparoscopic cystectomy.

E. Treatment with medroxyprogesterone acetate injections once a month for 6 months followed by surgical excision.

8. A 35-year-old woman complains of right-sided lower abdominal discomfort for one month. Her periods are regular. Abdominal and vaginal examinations are normal. Ultrasound scan reveals an unilocular, thin walled cyst, with no solid areas, measuring 4.5 cm in diameter in the right ovary.

What is the most appropriate management option?

A. Aspirate under ultrasound guidance.

B. Estimate CA-125 levels.

C. Perform a repeat ultrasound scan in 1 year.

D. Perform laparoscopic cystectomy.

E. Reassurance and no further follow-up.

9. A 55-year-old woman complains of right-sided lower abdominal discomfort for one month. She has reached menopause 2 years ago. Ultrasound scan reveals an unilocular, thin walled cyst with no solid areas, measuring 4.5 cm in diameter in the right ovary.

What is the next step in the management?

A. Aspirate under ultrasound guidance.

B. Estimate CA-125 levels.

C. Perform a repeat ultrasound scan in 4 months.

D. Perform laparoscopic cystectomy.

E. Reassurance and no further follow-up.

10. A 55-year-old woman complains of right-sided lower abdominal pain for one month. She has reached menopause 2 years ago. Ultrasound scan reveals an unilocular, thin-walled cyst with no solid areas, measuring 4.5 cm in diameter in the right ovary. CA-125 is 10 units/ml.

What is the next step in the management?

A. Aspirate under ultrasound guidance.

B. Perform a hysterectomy and bilateral salpingo-oophorectomy.

C. Perform a repeat ultrasound scan in 4 months.

D. Perform laparoscopic oophorectomy.

E. Reassurance and no further follow up.

11. A 57-year-old woman complains of right-sided lower abdominal pain for one month. She has reached menopause 5 years ago. Ultrasound scan reveals an unilocular, thin walled cyst with no solid areas, measuring 7.5 cm in diameter in the right ovary. CA-125 is 10 u/ml.

What is the next step in the management?

A. Aspirate under ultrasound guidance.

B. Perform a repeat ultrasound scan in 4 months.

C. Perform laparoscopic oophorectomy.

D. Perform a total abdominal hysterectomy and bilateral salpingo-oophorectomy.

E. Perform laparoscopic cystectomy.

12. A 40-year-old woman undergoes a total abdominal hysterectomy, bilateral salpingo oophorectomy and infracolic omentectomy for a malignant ovarian tumour. At surgery the tumour is found to be confined to one ovary without peritoneal deposits or ascites. Histology reveals a grade 1 mucinous tumour. The surface of the ovary is free of tumour. There are no malignant cells in the peritoneal washings.

What is the next step in the management?

A. Chemotherapy with cisplatin and taxane.

B. Chemotherapy with cisplatin.

C. Combined chemotherapy and radio-therapy.

D. No further treatment but regular follow-up for early detection of recu-rrence.

E. Radiotherapy

13. A 40-year-old woman undergoes a total abdominal hysterectomy, bilateral salpingo-oophorectomy and infracolic omentectomy for a stage IA malignant ovarian tumour. Histology reveals a grade 1 clear cell carcinoma.

What is the next step in the management?

A. Chemotherapy with cisplatin and taxane.

B. Chemotherapy with cisplatin.

C. Combined chemotherapy and radio-therapy.

D. Radiotherapy

E. Regular follow up for early detection of recurrence

ANSWERS AND EXPLANATIONS

Q. 1 (C)

This patient most probably has a benign dermoid cyst, because it is a smooth walled apparently benign cyst, with a hyperechoeic nodule less than 7 mm in diameter (Rokitansky nodule), thin echogenic bands caused by hair and no internal vascularity. The accepted treatment for a benign ovarian cyst in a premenopausal woman is ovarian cystectomy. Laparoscopy is safe in experienced hands, but care should be taken to avoid spilling of sebaceous material in a dermoid cyst. Oophorectomy is indicated if malignancy is suspected in a woman who desires future fertility. Total abdominal hysterectomy and bilateral salpingo-oophorectomy is indicated if malignancy is suspected in a woman who does not desire future fertility, or if the tumour has spread beyond the ovary in a young woman. Conservative treatment is contraindicated because the cyst is larger than 7 cm and has a solid component.

Q. 2 (A)

Since this woman is 49 years old and has a tumour with a solid component larger than 7 mm, hysterectomy and bilateral salpingo-oophorectomy is the best option, even though there are no other evidences of malignancy. However, CA-125 level should be done and the RMI should be calculated before the treatment is planned. If the RMI is more than 25 or if malignancy is suspected at operation, infracolic omentectomy and tumour staging should be done. Laparotomy is preferred to lapa-roscopy because of the presence of a solid nodule.

Q. 3 (D)

Laparotomy and right salpingo-oophorec-tomy is the most appropriate treatment, because this patient is 45 years of age and has a large, multilocular ovarian tumour. Even though the cyst is apparently benign, cystectomy should not be done, because the woman is 45 years of age and the cyst is large and multilocular. Recurrence can occur if mucinous material spills into the peritoneal cavity. A cystectomy should be done in a woman under the age of 40, after taking care to avoid spilling of cyst fluid into the peritoneal cavity. However, CA-125 levels should be done and the RMI should be calculated before surgery and the tumour and the peritoneal cavity should be inspected for signs of malignancy at the time of the operation. Laparoscopy is not recommended for cysts larger than 10 cm.

Q. 3a (C)

Since this woman is 30 years of age and has only 1 child, cystectomy should be done, after taking care to avoid spilling of cyst fluid into the peritoneal cavity. However, CA-125 levels should be done and the RMI should be calculated before surgery and the tumour and the peritoneal cavity should be inspected for signs of malignancy at the time of the operation. Laparoscopy is not recommended for cysts larger than 10 cm. Oophorectomy is indicated only if malignancy is suspected. Hysterectomy is indicated in a younger woman only if malignancy is confirmed.

Q. 4 (B)

This patient has a stage IIB tumour for which the accepted treatment is total abdominal hysterectomy and bilateral salpingo-oophorectomy with infracolic omentectomy followed by chemotherapy. If the tumour is confined to one ovary and the stage is IA, unilateral salpingo-oophorectomy, infracolic omentectomy, full thickness biopsy of the other ovary and surgical staging would be the most appropriate procedure, as this patient will desire future fertility. Preoperative chemotherapy is indicated only in extensive tumours where initial debulking is not possible.

Q. 5 (B)

Since serum alpha-fetoprotein levels are elevated and the woman is young, she most probably has an endodermal sinus cell tumour or less commonly another germ cell tumour, such as an embryonal cell carcinoma, immature teratoma, or a polyembryoma. These germ cell tumours are sensitive to chemotherapy

with bleomycin, etoposide, and cisplatin (BEP) or a combination of cisplatin, vinblastine, and bleomycin. Therefore, the best treatment option in a young woman with a germ cell tumour, who wishes to preserve fertility, is conservative surgery followed by chemotherapy.

This woman has a stage IA tumour. Therefore, the first line therapy is unilateral salpingo-oophorectomy, infracolic omentectomy and full thickness biopsy of the other ovary. Laparoscopic surgery is not recommended as tumour tissue can spill to the peritoneal cavity. If the woman had completed the family, the best option would be total abdominal hysterectomy and bilateral salpingo-oophorectomy with infracolic omentectomy. Ovarian cystectomy is never done for the treatment of an ovarian tumour if malignancy is suspected.

Q. 6 (D)

Since this patient who has an ovarian tumour has developed sudden onset of pain and vomiting torsion has to be suspected. The ovarian cyst is most probably a dermoid cyst because it has benign features (thin intact capsule and localised to the ovary) with a solid focus less than 7 mm and thin hair like echogenic bands. Surgery should be done as soon as possible if torsion is suspected, because the ovary cannot be saved if gangrene occurs. Since this woman is very young and desires future fertility, the best treatment option is to perform an ovarian cystectomy. However, oophorectomy should be done if the ovary is gangrenous, or if malignancy is suspected at operation. Cystectomy by laparoscopy is the best option, but care should be taken to avoid spilling sebaceous material into the peritoneal cavity, if it is a dermoid cyst.

Q. 7 (D)

A diagnosis of an endometriotic cyst can be made because the patient is infertile with dysmenorrhoea, dyspareunia and short menstrual cycles. Also the cyst has echogenic fluid. Surgery is the first line treatment as the cyst is larger than 5 cm and the patient desires fertility. Medical treatment is not recommended as she desires fertility as soon as possible.

Q. 8 (E)

Since the woman is premenopausal and the cyst is less than 5 cm and appears benign on ultrasound scanning, she should be reassured and discharged from the clinic. If the diameter of the cyst is between 5 and 7 cm, a repeat scan is done in one year. Laparoscopic cystectomy is the treatment of choice for benign ovarian cysts which are larger than 7 cm. Aspiration is not recommend as refilling can occur.

Q. 9 (B)

When a postmenopausal woman is found to have an apparently benign ovarian cyst on the ultrasound scan, the next step in the management is to perform CA-125 levels, as the RMI should be calculated. Serum CA-125 is raised in over 80% of ovarian cancer cases and if a cut-off value of 30 units/ml is used, the test has a sensitivity of 81% and specificity of 75%. Further management depends on the CA-125 level and the RMI.

Q. 10 (C)

Simple, unilateral, unilocular ovarian cysts, less than 5 cm in diameter, have a low risk of malignancy. It is recommended that if serum CA-125 levels are within the normal range, they can be managed conservatively, as more than 50% of these cysts will resolve spontaneously within three months. A repeat ultrasound scan should be performed in four months as this woman is postmenopausal.

Q. 11 (C)

Simple, unilateral, unilocular ovarian cysts, with normal CA-125 levels have a low risk of malignancy. However, surgery is indicated because the woman is postmenopausal and the cyst is larger than 5 cm. The main reason to perform surgery in a postmenopausal woman with an ovarian cyst is to exclude malignancy and to perform a full staging procedure. Laparoscopic surgery is performed only if there is a low risk of malignancy. Laparo-scopic oophorectomy is the best option for this woman, as she has a thin-walled cyst with no septa or solid areas giving an ultrasound score of 0 and normal CA-125 levels. Ovarian cystectomy is not performed in postmenopausal women.

Q. 12 (D)

This woman has a stage IA grade 1 muci-nous tumour. Patients with stage IA grade 1 and stage IB grade 1, serous, mucinous, endometrioid and Brenner tumours can be treated with surgery alone. She only needs regular follow-up.

Q. 13 (A)

This woman has a stage IA clear cell carcinoma. Clear cell carcinomas have a worse prognosis in stage I and should be considered for chemotherapy at all stages. Therefore, she needs chemotherapy with taxane and cisplatin, which are the standard chemotherapeutic agents used for malignant ovarian tumours.

REFERENCES

- Ovarian Cysts in Postmenopausal Women, RCOG Guideline No. 34, October 2003, Reviewed 2010.
- Management of Suspected Ovarian Masses in Premenopausal Women, Green-top Guideline No. 62, RCOG/BSGE Joint Guideline I, November 2011.
- Ovarian cancer: Recognition and initial management, NICE Guidelines [CG122] Published date: April 2011.

7

Cervical Intraepithelial Neoplasia

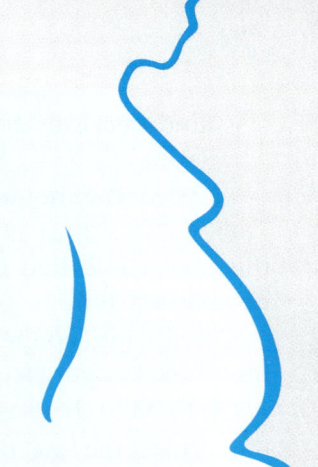

SQUAMOUS METAPLASIA AND DYSPLASIA

- Ectocervix is the visible part of the cervix while the endocervix is invisible and lies proximal to the external os.
- Ectocervix is covered by pink stratified squamous epithelium, consisting of multiple layers of cells. Reddish columnar epithelium consisting of a single layer of cells line the endocervix.
- The squamocolumnar junction (SCJ) is at the external os during infancy, but as the cervix increases in volume during puberty and in pregnancy, the SCJ spreads out onto the ectocervix.
- An ectropion occurs due to the growth of the columnar epithelium onto the ectocervix, when rapid growth and enlargement of the cervix occurs under the influence of oestrogen, during the reproductive life. It is commonly seen during pregnancy, but does not occur after menopause.
- Replacement of the everted columnar epithelium on the ectocervix, by a newly formed squamous epithelium from the subcolumnar reserve cells, is called squamous metaplasia.
- The transformation zone is the region of the cervix where squamous metaplasia takes place.
- The transformation zone should be identified during colposcopy, as almost all manifestations of cervical carcinogenesis occur in this zone.
- Disruption of the process of metaplasia by external influences can lead to disordered squamous epithelium called dysplastic epithelium.
- The nuclei of dysplastic cells are larger and more variable in size and shape. They divide more actively and lack the normal maturation of healthy squamous epithelial cells.
- Dysplasia is referred to as cervical intraepithelial neoplasia (CIN).

BETHESDA SYSTEM OF CLASSIFICATION OF CERVICAL INTRAEPITHELIAL LESIONS

- Negative for intraepithelial lesion or malignancy
- Epithelial cell abnormalities
  - Squamous cell
  - Atypical squamous cells of undetermined significance (ASC-US)
  - Atypical squamous cells—cannot exclude HSIL (ASC-H)
  - Low-grade squamous intraepithelial lesion (LSIL)
  - High-grade squamous intraepithelial lesion (HSIL)
  - Squamous cell carcinoma
- Glandular
  - Atypical glandular cells (AGC)

- Endocervical adenocarcinoma *in situ* (AIS)
- Adenocarcinoma

Dysplasia that is seen on a biopsy of the cervix is called cervical intraepithelial neoplasia (CIN).

Cervical intraepithelial neoplasia is grouped into three categories:

- CIN I: Mild dysplasia (LSIL).
  - This is the least risky type with only mild dysplasia, or abnormal cell growth. It involves the basal 1/3 of the epithelium.
  - This usually corresponds to infection with HPV, and may be cleared by the immune response, though it can take several years to clear.
- CIN II: Moderate to marked dysplasia (HSIL).
  - The changes involve the basal 2/3 of the epithelium.
- CIN III: Severe dysplasia to carcinoma *in situ* (HSIL).
  - The changes are found in more than 2/3 of the epithelium and may involve the full thickness.
  - The lesion is regarded as cervical carcinoma *in situ*.

Screening Guidelines for Cervical Intraepithelial Neoplasia

- Cervical cancer screening should be commenced at 21 years of age (USA). However, different ages are advised in different countries. In UK screening is commenced at 25 years while in Sri Lanka it is commenced at 35 years. Screening should be commenced about 10 years after commencing sexual intercourse.
- A Pap test should be performed every 3 years in women between the ages of 21 and 29. Testing for HPV is indicated only if the Pap test result is abnormal.
- A Pap test and an HPV test should be performed every 5 years in women between

the ages of 30 and 65. However, a Pap test alone may be performed every 3 years.

- Cervical cancer screening is not indicated in women over age 65 years who have been previously screened regularly with normal results. However, women who have cervical pre-cancer should continue to be screened.
- Women who have undergone a total hysterectomy should not be screened, if they do not have a previous history of cervical cancer or pre-cancer.
- Women who have been given the HPV vaccine should still follow the screening program recommended for their age group.
- Women with HIV infection, organ transplant, or exposure to the drug DES are at a higher risk of cervical cancer and should be screened more often.

FURTHER EVALUATION OF ABNORMAL CYTOLOGY RESULTS

Cytology-negative, HPV-positive Test Results

- The risk of developing CIN 2–3+ is about 4%.
- Therefore, colposcopy is not recommended.
- Cytology and HPV testing should be repeated in 12 months, to allow time for resolution of a transient HPV infection.
- Colposcopy is done only if the follow-up results are abnormal (i.e. HPV-positive or ASC-US or higher-grade cytology results).

Atypical Squamous Cells of Unknown Significance (ASC-US)

- Test for high-risk HPV types. If the test is positive, colposcopy is done.
- If the HPV test is negative, the risk of having CIN 2–3+ is less than 2% and they can be referred for follow-up.
- Follow-up include repeat cytology and HPV testing in 1 year.
- Colposcopy is done if HPV testing is positive or cytology is ASC-US or greater on follow-up.

- Adolescents have a very low risk of invasive cancer and the likelihood of HPV clearance is very high. Therefore, cytology testing is performed at 6 and 12 months or a single HPV test is performed at 12 months in adolescents with ASC and HPV-positive test results. Colposcopy is performed only for an abnormal cytology result or positive HPV test result during follow-up.

Atypical Squamous Cells—Cannot Exclude High-grade Squamous Intraepithelial Lesion (ASC-H)

- The incidence of CIN 2, 3 is as high as 50%.
- Therefore, colposcopy is recommended.
- HPV testing for women with ASC-H is not included in the guideline but a negative test is reassuring.
- Cytology testing at 6 and 12 months or an HPV DNA test at 12 months is performed if colposcopy reveals CIN 1 or normal or results. Excision is not indicated for these women.

LSIL

- The risk of CIN 2–3+ at initial colposcopy following a LSIL result is between 15 and 30%.
- Therefore, colposcopy is performed for further investigation of LSIL.
- Cytology testing at 6 and 12 months or an HPV DNA test at 12 months is performed if colposcopy reveals CIN 1 or normal results. Excision is not indicated for these women.
- Adolescents with LSIL have a very low risk of invasive cancer and the likelihood of HPV clearance is very high. Therefore, immediate colposcopy is not recommended and they are followed up in a similar manner as adolescents with ASC HPV-positive results.

HSIL

- CIN 2 or CIN 3 occurs in about 70% of women with high grade squamous intraepithelial lesions (HSIL), and 1 to 2% have invasive cancer.

- Colposcopy and biopsy of visible lesions is recommended. Biopsy may be performed from an abnormal area detected on colposcopy. Biopsy is essential when a visual diagnosis of CIN 2 or CIN 3 is made
- CIN 2 and CIN 3 are potential cancer precursors, although CIN 2 can undergo spontaneous regression.
- Non-pregnant patients with CIN 2 and CIN 3 require immediate treatment with excision.
- Follow-up similar to CIN 1 may be considered in adolescents with CIN 2, as they have a low risk of invasive cancer and a high incidence of spontaneous clearance. Therefore, treatment of adolescents with CIN 2 may be individualized.
- Hysterectomy is not regarded as the first line treatment for patients with CIN 2 or CIN 3 in the absence of other indications. Hysterectomy is performed for persistent or recurrent CIN 2 or CIN 3, or when a repeat excision is indicated but technically not feasible. Invasive cancer should be ruled out before hysterectomy is performed.

TREATMENT

- Cryotherapy
  - Cryotherapy can be performed if the entire lesion and the squamocolumnar junction are visible, and the lesion does not cover more than three quarters of the ectocervix.
  - Cryotherapy is not performed if the lesion extends beyond the cryoprobe, or into the endocervical canal, or when there is suspicion of malignancy.
- Loop electrosurgical excision
  - This method is preferred for CIN 2 and CIN 3 because histological examination is possible.
  - It is also possible to determine whether the entire lesion has been removed.
- Cold knife conisation is carried out if the above procedures are not available. This

procedure has the disadvantages of needing hospital admission and occurrence of bleeding.

Prevention of Cervical Cancer

Cervical cancer can be prevented by vaccinating girls between the ages of 9–13 years (at least by 15 years) with 2 doses of HPV vaccine 6 months apart. Vaccination should be done before commencing sexual intercourse.

SUMMARY

- Colposcopy is recommended for adult women with:
  - a low-grade squamous intraepithelial lesion,
  - atypical glandular cells,
  - high-grade squamous intraepithelial lesion,
  - atypical squamous cells—cannot exclude high-grade intraepithelial neoplasia.
  - ASC-US who are HPV DNA positive
- Cervical intraepithelial neoplasia, grade 1 is managed conservatively in adult women.
- Cervical intraepithelial neoplasia, grades 2 and 3 require immediate treatment.
- Colposcopy and endocervical curettage is indicated in women with AGC and AIS. HPV DNA testing or repeat cytology is not suitable for the management of those with AGC and AIS.
- Colposcopy is performed for pregnant women with low-grade squamous intra-

epithelial lesion and high-grade squamous intraepithelial lesion. However, further treatment of the former is postponed until six weeks postpartum. Treatment during pregnancy is indicated only for invasive carcinoma.

WHO recommends a screen- and- treat-strategy for middle and low income developing countries. This protocol is cheap, easy to perform and does not need expertise. This prevents women being lost to follow-up as they are treated immediately.

The screening strategies
- Screen with HPV test alone.
- Screen with HPV test and visual inspection with acetic acid. (VIA)
- Screen with VIA alone.

Screen positive women are treated immediately with cryotherapy or with LEEP if they are not eligible for cryotherapy.

REFERENCES

- Carrie A. Morantz, Am Fam Physician. ACOG Releases Guidelines for Management of Abnormal Cervical Cytology and Histology, Feb 2006 15; 73(4):719–729.
- 2012 Updated ASCCP Consensus Guidelines for the Management of Abnormal Cervical Cancer Screening Tests and Cancer Precursors.
- Comprehensive Cervical Cancer Control, A Guide to Essential Practice, 2nd ed., World Health Organisation.

QUESTIONS

1. **A 30-year-old woman undergoes cervical cancer screening. The report states the presence of atypical squamous cells of undetermined significance.**
   What is the next step in the management?
   A. Perform colposcopy.
   B. Perform cryotherapy.
   C. Repeat the smear in 2 years.
   D. Repeat the smear in 6 months.
   E. Test for infection with high risk HPV types.

2. **A 30-year-old woman undergoes cervical cancer screening. The report states the presence of atypical squamous**

cells of undetermined significance. On subsequent testing she is found to be negative for infection with high risk HPV types.

What is the next step in the management?

A. Perform colposcopy.

B. Perform knife cone biopsy.

C. Repeat the HPV tests in 6 months.

D. Repeat the smear and HPV test in 1 year.

E. Repeat the smear in 2 years.

2a. A 30-year-old woman undergoes cervical cancer screening. The report states the presence of atypical squamous cells of undetermined significance. On subsequent testing she is found to be positive for infection with high risk HPV types. What is the next step in the management?

A. Perform colposcopy.

B. Perform cryotherapy.

C. Perform loop electro-surgical excision.

D. Repeat the smear and HPV test in 1 year.

E. Repeat the smear in 2 years.

3. A 30-year-old woman is found to have a low grade squamous intraepithelial lesion on routine cervical cancer screening.

What is the next step in the management?

A. Perform colposcopy.

B. Perform loop electrosurgical excision.

C. Perform visual inspection with acetic acid.

D. Repeat the smear in 2 years if there is no HPV infection.

E. Repeat the smear in 6 months.

4. A 35-year-old multiparous woman is found to have a high grade squamous intraepithelial lesion on routine cervical cancer screening. Colposcopy and biopsy reveals the presence of CIN 2.

What is the next step in the management?

A. Perform loop electrosurgical excision.

B. Perform a cone biopsy.

C. Perform a hysterectomy.

D. Repeat the smear in 2 years if there is no HPV infection.

E. Repeat the smear in 6 months.

5. A 35-year-old woman attends the clinic with a complaint of vaginal discharge. On examination a small ulcer is found on the anterior lip of the cervix.

What is the next step in the management?

A. Perform a cervical smear.

B. Perform a cone biopsy.

C. Perform a wedge biopsy of the lesion.

D. Perform colposcopy and directed biopsy.

E. Test for high risk HPV types.

6. A 20-year-old woman is found to have a low grade squamous intraepithelial lesion on routine cervical cancer screening.

What is the next step in the management?

A. Perform colposcopy and loop electro-surgical excision.

B. Perform colposcopy.

C. Perform visual inspection with acetic acid.

D. Repeat the smear and HPV test in 1 year.

E. Repeat the smear in 2 years if there is no HPV infection.

7. A 20-year-old woman is found to have a high grade squamous intraepithelial lesion on routine cervical cancer screening.

What is the next step in the management?

A. Perform a cone biopsy.

B. Perform colposcopy and loop electro-surgical excision.

C. Perform colposcopy.

D. Repeat the smear and HPV test in 1 year.

E. Repeat the smear in 2 years if there is no HPV infection.

8. A 20-year-old woman is found to have a high grade squamous intraepithelial lesion on routine cervical cancer screening. Colposcopy and biopsy reveals a histological diagnosis of CIN 2.

   What is the next step in the management?

   A. Perform a cone biopsy.
   B. Perform colposcopy and loop electro-surgical excision.
   C. Perform cytology and colposcopy every 6 months for 24 months.
   D. Repeat the smear and HPV test in 1 year.
   E. Repeat the smear in 2 years if there is no HPV infection.

9. A 35-year-old woman is found to have atypical glandular cells on routine cervical cancer screening.

   What is the next step in the management?

   A. Perform a cone biopsy.
   B. Perform colposcopy and endocervical curettage.
   C. Repeat the smear in 2 years if there is no HPV infection.
   D. Repeat the smear in 6 months.
   E. Test for infection with high risk HPV types.

ANSWERS AND EXPLANATIONS

Q. 1 (E)

Q. 2 (D)

Q. 2a (A)

Explanation for questions 1, 2 and 2a

If atypical squamous cells of undetermined significance are found in the cervical smear, the next step in the management is to test for high risk HPV types. If the HPV test is negative the woman can be reassured that her risk of having CIN 2–3+ is less than 2%, and can be referred for follow-up. The smear should be repeated in 6 months and 1 year and the HPV test is repeated in 1 year. Colposcopy is done if the woman is positive for infection with high risk HPV types at initial testing, or if repeat HPV test is positive or cytology is ASC-US or greater on follow-up. Treatment is not indicated for ASC-US.

Q. 3 (A)

Detection of CIN 2–3 at colposcopy in LSIL is between 15 and 30% in most studies. Therefore, colposcopy is recommended as the first step for evaluation of LSIL. Colposcopy is preferable to VIA as accurate evaluation is possible. Follow-up of a colposcopy result of CIN 1 or normal should include cytological testing at 6 and 12 months or a HPV DNA test at 12 months, rather than excision.

Q. 4 (A)

CIN 2 and CIN 3 are regarded as potential cancer precursors. However, a significant number of patients with CIN 2 can undergo spontaneous regression. Immediate treatment of CIN 2 and CIN 3 with excision or ablation is recommended in non-pregnant patients. Therefore, the next step in the management is to perform loop electrosurgical excision. This can be performed in the outpatient department and is preferred over cone biopsy, which is a bloody procedure which needs hospital admission. Cryotherapy is also an option but a specimen cannot be obtained for histological examination. Hysterectomy is not regarded as the first line treatment for patients with CIN 2 or CIN 3 in the absence of other indications. Hysterectomy is performed for persistent or recurrent CIN 2 or CIN 3, or when a repeat excision is indicated but technically not feasible. Invasive cancer should be excluded before hysterectomy is performed.

Q. 5 (C)

Cervical smear test and testing for high risk HPV types are screening tests for cervical cancer, which are done in the absence of a visible lesion. Colposcopy is done for investigation of a squamous intraepithelial lesion and cone biopsy is done for the treatment of CIN 1 or CIN 2, in the absence of a visible lesion. When there is a visible lesion the first step in the management is to perform a wedge biopsy from the lesion.

Q. 6 (D)

Adolescents with any cytological or histological diagnosis except cervical intraepithelial neoplasia, grade 3 and adenocarcinoma *in situ* are best treated conservatively. Adolescents with LSIL results are followed up without immediate colposcopy, because clearance of HPV is high and cancer rates are extremely low. Therefore, they are monitored with cytology testing at 6 and 12 months or with a single HPV test at 12 months.

Q. 7 (C)

Q. 8 (C)

Explanation for questions 7 and 8

Colposcopy is the next step in the management in adolescents with HSIL, but imme-diate excision is not recommended if CIN 3 is not found. If CIN 2 is found, observation with cytology and histology every 6 months for 24 months is preferred. Treatment with excision is recommended if CIN 3 is found, or if colposcopy is unsatisfactory or if HSIL persists for 24 months. It is unacceptable to perform an excisional procedure without histological confirmation because of the risk of future obstetric complications.

Q. 9 (B)

Colposcopy and endocervical curettage is indicated in women with AGC and AIS. HPV DNA testing or repeat cytology is not suitable for the management of those with AGC and AIS.

REFERENCES

- John W. Sellors. Colposcopy and Treatment of Cervical Intra-epithelial Neoplasia: A Beginners' Manual.

- American Society for Colposcopy and Cervical Pathology—Algorithms Updated Consensus Guidelines for Managing Abnormal Cervical Cancer Screening Tests and Cancer Precursors.

Cervical Carcinoma

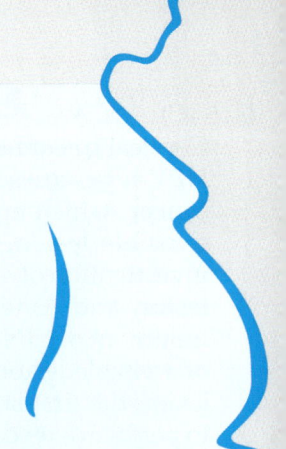

- There are two main types of cervical cancer—squamous cell carcinoma and adenocarcinoma.
- A premalignant phase occurs in squamous cell carcinoma. It precedes the onset of the cancer by about 10 years.
- Cervical cytology is designed to detect squamous abnormalities of the cervix, but also detects some glandular abnormalities.
- With regular, frequent screening it is possible to detect and treat most squamous cancers at the premalignant stage.
- Due to regular screening programs the incidence of cervical cancer has fallen. The benefit is more for squamous cancers than for adenocarcinoma.
- Depending on several factors and the location of the infection, CIN can start in any of the three stages, and can either progress, or regress.

HPV types 16 and 18 are associated with cervical cancer, but many other types are also found. A HPV DNA test can identify the high-risk types of HPV linked to cancer and may be carried out:

- once in 5 years in the regular screening program for women over age 30.
- in the further investigation of women who have a slightly abnormal smear test result.

Risk factors for cervical cancer include:

- increased parity
- sexual promiscuity

- early marriage and young age at time of first sexual intercourse
- low socioeconomic status
- smoking
- long-term use of oral contraceptives.

SYMPTOMS

- May have no symptoms
- Irregular bleeding
- Blood stained vaginal discharge
- Postcoital bleeding
- Dyspareunia
- Pelvic pain

DIAGNOSIS

- Is by histological examination of a biopsy specimen.
- Early stages up to stage IA2 are diagnosed by cervical cytology followed by colposcopy and biopsy.
- Direct biopsy of a visible lesion is done from stage IB onwards.
- MRI scan may be necessary to stage the disease accurately and to determine the extent of spread.

FIGO STAGING OF CERVICAL CARCINOMA

Stage I

Carcinoma is confined to the cervix. Extension to the uterine corpus is disregarded. Stages

IA1 and IA2 are diagnosed on microscopic examination of removed tissue, preferably a cone, which must include the entire lesion.

- **Stage IA:** Invasive cancer identified only microscopically. Invasion is limited to a maximum depth of 5 mm and a width of 7 mm.
- **Stage IA1:** Measured stromal invasion is less than 3 mm in depth and 7 mm in width.
- **Stage IA2:** Measured stromal invasion is greater than 3 mm but not greater than 5 mm in depth and no wider than 7 mm in diameter.
- **Stage IB:** Clinical lesions confined to the cervix or preclinical lesions greater than stage IA. All gross visible lesions are stage IB cancers even if the invasion is minimal.
- **Stage IB1:** Visible lesions smaller than 4 cm in size.
- **Stage IB2:** Visible lesions larger than 4 cm in size.

Stage II

Stage II tumours extend beyond the cervix, but do not extend into the pelvic wall. The tumour involves the upper two-thirds of the vagina, but not the lower third.

- **Stage IIA:** There is no parametrial involvement. The lesion has spread to the upper two-thirds of the vagina.
- **Stage IIB:** The lesion has spread to the parametrium but not into the pelvic sidewall.

Stage III

Stage III tumour extends into the lateral pelvic wall. On rectal examination, a cancer-free space is not found between the tumour and the lateral pelvic wall. The tumour has spread to the lower third of the vagina. All cases with hydronephrosis or a non-functioning kidney fall into stage III.

- **Stage IIIA:** The lateral pelvic wall is not involved but the tumour has spread to the lower third of the vagina.
- **Stage IIIB:** Extension into the lateral pelvic wall or presence of hydronephrosis or non-functioning kidney.

Stage IV

Stage IV tumour has spread beyond the true pelvis or has involved the mucosa of the bladder and/or rectum.

- **Stage IVA:** The tumour has spread into adjacent pelvic organs.
- **Stage IVB:** Spread to distant organs.

TREATMENT

Stage IA1—preclinical invasive disease which invades to a depth of less than 3 mm and a width of less than 7 mm.

- Removal of pelvic lymph nodes is not required for FIGO IA1 disease.
- Standard treatment for IA1 disease is simple hysterectomy if fertility is not an issue. However, regular follow-up with vault smears is necessary.
- If fertility conservation is required, cold knife conisation or loop electrosurgical excision and follow-up is adequate. The margins of the cone should not contain tumour cells.

Stage IA2—preclinical invasive disease which invades to a depth between 3 and 5 mm and a width of less than 7 mm.

- Removal of pelvic lymph nodes is recommended for FIGO IA2 disease.
- The standard treatment is modified radical hysterectomy (Piver type 2). This includes dissection of the ureters, ligation of the uterine arteries medial to the ureters, excision of the uterosacral ligaments midway from the sacral insertion, resection of the medial half of the cardinal ligaments and removal of the upper third of the vagina and pelvic lymphadenectomy. If the nodes contain cancer cells, postoperative radiotherapy and chemotherapy with cisplatin is necessary.
- Women who desire fertility are offered radical trachelectomy. This involves vaginal resection of the cervix, the upper 1 to 2 cm of the vaginal cuff and the medial portions of the cardinal and uterosacral ligaments. The cervix is transected at the lower uterine

segment and a prophylactic cerclage is placed at the time of surgery. Radical trachelectomy must be combined with pelvic lymph node dissection for IA2 and IB1 disease. Follow-up is with Pap smears performed at 4 and 10 months and annually if these two smears are normal.

- External beam radiation therapy to the pelvis and brachytherapy is recommended for patients who are medically unfit for surgery or refuse surgery.

Stage IB1—clinical lesion confined to the cervix but smaller than 4 cm.

- The standard treatment is radical hysterectomy (type 3). This includes complete dissection of the ureters, ligation of the uterine arteries close to the hypogastric region, excision of the uterosacral ligaments at the sacral insertion, excision of the cardinal ligaments close to the lateral pelvic wall, removal of the upper half of the vagina and pelvic lymph node dissection. If the nodes contain cancer cells postoperative radiotherapy and chemotherapy with cisplatin is necessary.

- Radical trachelectomy with pelvic lymph node dissection may be considered if the patient still wants to preserve her fertility.
- Another option is chemoradiotherapy. Both brachytherapy and external beam radiation therapy is used together with chemotherapy.

Stage IB2—clinical lesion confined to the cervix but larger than 4 cm.

- The standard treatment is chemotherapy with cisplatin or cisplatin and 5 fluorouracil with radiation therapy (chemoradiotherapy). Both external beam radiation and brachytherapy are used. Brachytherapy is short wave radiotherapy delivered by the insertion of applicators into the uterus via the vagina.
- Radical hysterectomy is not the best option if the tumour measures more than 4 cm, because of the increased likelihood of needing postoperative chemoradiotherapy.
- Generally chemoradiotherapy is used to treat women with FIGO IB2, IIA, IIB, IIIA, IIIB and IVA disease. Surgery is not offered because of the significant risk of positive margins and positive nodes.

QUESTIONS

1. **A 35-year-old multiparous woman is found to have preclinical invasive disease of the cervix penetrating to a depth of 2 mm with a width of 5 mm. She has no fertility wishes.**

   What is the most appropriate treatment?
   A. Knife cone biopsy.
   B. Loop electrosurgical excision of the transformation zone.
   C. Repeat colposcopy in three months.
   D. Total hysterectomy.
   E. Wertheim's hysterectomy.

2. **A 25-year-old woman with one child has preclinical invasive disease of the cervix penetrating to a depth of 2 mm with a** width of 5 mm. **She wishes to preserve her fertility.**

   What is the most appropriate treatment?
   A. Knife cone biopsy.
   B. Loop electrosurgical excision of the transformation zone.
   C. Repeat colposcopy in three months.
   D. Total hysterectomy.
   E. Wertheim's hysterectomy.

3. **A 42-year-old multiparous woman is found to have preclinical invasive disease of the cervix penetrating to a depth of 4 mm with a width of 7 mm.**

   What is the most appropriate treatment?

A. Chemoradiotherapy.

B. Modified radical hysterectomy.

C. Radical trachelectomy.

D. Knife cone biopsy.

E. Total hysterectomy.

4. **A 30-year-old woman with one child is found to have preclinical invasive disease of the cervix penetrating to a depth of 4 mm with a width of 7 mm. She wishes to preserve her fertility.**

   What is the most appropriate treatment?

   A. Chemoradiotherapy.

   B. Knife cone biopsy.

   C. Radical trachelectomy with pelvic lymph node dissection.

   D. Radical trachelectomy.

   E. Radiotherapy.

5. **A 30-year-old woman with one child is found to have a visible cervical lesion measuring 2 cm. Biopsy of the lesion reveals a squamous carcinoma of the cervix. The lesion is confined to the cervix. She wishes to preserve her fertility.**

   What is the most appropriate treatment?

   A. Chemoradiotherapy.

   B. Knife cone biopsy

   C. Radical trachelectomy.

   D. Radical trachelectomy with pelvic lymph node dissection.

   E. Radiotherapy.

6. **A 45-year-old woman is found to have a cervical lesion measuring 2 cm. Biopsy of**
the lesion reveals a squamous carcinoma of the cervix. The lesion is confined to the cervix.

What is the most appropriate treatment?

A. Chemoradiotherapy.

B. Radical hysterectomy.

C. Radical trachelectomy with pelvic lymph node dissection.

D. Radiotherapy.

E. Total abdominal hysterectomy.

7. **A 30-year-old woman with one child is found to have a cervical lesion measuring 4 cm. Biopsy of the lesion reveals a squamous carcinoma of the cervix. The lesion is confined to the cervix.**

   What is the most appropriate treatment?

   A. Neoadjuvant chemotherapy followed by radical hysterectomy.

   B. Radiotherapy.

   C. Radical trachelectomy with pelvic lymph node dissection.

   D. Chemoradiotherapy.

   E. Radical hysterectomy.

8. **A 42-year-old woman is found to have a cervical carcinoma extending to the upper part of the vagina and the medial part of the parametrium.**

   What is the best treatment option?

   A. Radiotherapy.

   B. Wertheim's hysterectomy.

   C. Chemoradiotherapy.

   D. Total abdominal hysterectomy and dissection of the pelvic lymph nodes.

   E. Chemotherapy.

ANSWERS AND EXPLANATIONS

Q. 1 (D)

This woman has stage IA1 carcinoma of the cervix. Standard treatment for stage IA1 disease is simple hysterectomy if fertility is not an issue. However, regular follow-up with vault smears is necessary. Wertheim's hysterectomy or removal of pelvic lymph nodes is not recommended for FIGO IA1 disease. If fertility conservation is required loop electrosurgical excision of the transformation zone and follow-up is adequate. The margins of the removed tissue should not contain tumour cells. Cold knife conisation is an option.

Q. 2 (B)

This woman has stage IA1 carcinoma of the cervix. As fertility conservation is required loop electrosurgical (LEEP) excision of the transformation zone and follow-up is adequate. The margins of the removed tissue should not contain tumour cells. LEEP is a better option than knife cone biopsy, as it can be done as an outpatient procedure and does not cause much bleeding. Repeat colposcopy is not indicated before treatment as invasive disease will not regress.

Q. 3 (B)

This woman has stage IA2 carcinoma of the cervix. The standard treatment is modified radical hysterectomy (Piver type 2 operation). This operation requires more extensive dissection than the extrafascial hysterectomy. The medial half of the uterosacral ligaments and the cardinal ligaments are removed. The uterine artery is ligated just medial to the point at which it crosses the ureter. 1–2 cm portion of the upper vagina is removed and pelvic and para-aortic lymphadenectomy is performed. External beam radiation therapy to the pelvis and brachytherapy is recommended for patients who are medically unfit for surgery or refuse surgery. Total hysterectomy alone is not carried out as pelvic lymph node dissection is recommended for stage IA2 disease. Radical trachelectomy with pelvic lymph node dissection is an alternative for those who wish to retain their fertility.

Q. 4 (C)

This woman has stage IA2 carcinoma of the cervix. Women, who desire fertility, are offered radical trachelectomy with pelvic lymph node dissection.

Q. 5 (D)

This woman has stage IB1 disease. Radical trachelectomy with pelvic lymph node dissection is an option, after coun-selling, if the woman still desires to preserve her fertility.

Q. 6 (B)

This woman has a stage IB1 carcinoma of the cervix. The standard treatment is type 3 radical hysterectomy. As much parametrial tissue as possible is removed. The uterosacral ligaments are divided close to their origin from the sacrum. The cardinal ligaments are excised as widely as possible, after ligating the uterine artery at its origin, where it branches off the hypogastric artery. The superior vesical artery should be preserved. A 2–3 cm portion of the upper vagina is removed and pelvic and para-aortic lymphadenectomy is performed. Chemoradiotherapy is also a treatment option.

Q. 7 (D)

This woman has a stage IB2 carcinoma of the cervix. The standard treatment is chemotherapy with cisplatin or cisplatin and 5 fluorouracil with radiation therapy (chemoradiotherapy). Both external beam radiation and brachytherapy are used. Radical hysterectomy with pelvic lymph node dissection and postoperative chemoradiotherapy is an optional method of treatment. Neoadjuvant chemotherapy (three rapidly delivered courses of platinum-based chemotherapy) followed by radical hysterectomy and pelvic lymphadenectomy is also an option.

Q. 8 (C)

This woman has stage IIB cervical carcinoma which is best treated by chemoradiotherapy.

REFERENCE

- J.L. Benedet, H. Bender, H. Jones III, H.Y.S. Ngan, S. Pecorelli. Staging Classifications and Clinical Practice Guidelines of Gynaecologic Cancers, FIGO Committee on Gynaecologic Oncology.

9

Infections in Gynaecology

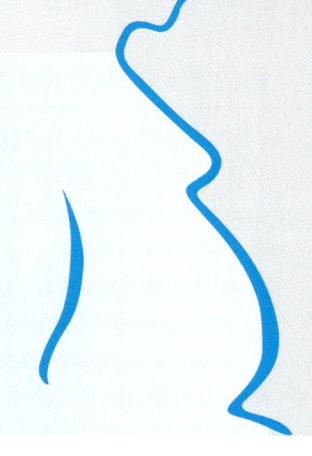

PHYSIOLOGICAL DISCHARGE— LEUCORRHOEA

Normal vaginal discharge is non-offensive, non-pruritic, white and becomes yellowish on contact with air, due to oxidation. It may increase at mid-cycle and before menstruation.

VAGINAL INFECTIONS

CANDIDIASIS

- Is caused by *Candida albicans* which is a gram-positive yeast.
- It infects the stratified squamous epithelium of the vagina.
- It does not cause pelvic inflammatory disease.
- It is a commensal organism and is not sexually transmitted.
- The classical presentation is itching and soreness of the vagina and vulva, with a curdy, white discharge, which becomes adherent to the vaginal epithelium as white plaques.

Predisposing Factors

- Immunosuppression—HIV, immunosuppressive therapy, e.g. steroids.
- Diabetes mellitus.
- Vaginal douching, bubble bath, shower gel, tight clothing.

- Increased oestrogen—pregnancy, high-dose combined oral contraceptive pill.
- Underlying dermatosis, e.g. eczema.
- Broad-spectrum antibiotic therapy.

Diagnosis

- The condition can be diagnosed clinically by the presence of the classical symptoms of pruritus and white, thick, vaginal discharge.
- Diagnosis is usually confirmed by microscopy of the vaginal discharge.
  - A direct smear will show budding yeast cells.
  - A gram stained smear shows gram-positive yeasts.
  - The diagnosis can be further confirmed by culture in the Feinberg Whittington Medium.

Treatment

- Women with asymptomatic Candida colonization do not require treatment as the organism is a commensal.
- Topical treatment by inserting vaginal tablets is more effective than systemic treatment.
- A single dose of treatment with clotrimazole 500 mg is adequate.
- If oral treatment is required at the time of menstruation or in an unmarried woman, a single 150 mg tablet of fluconazole is effective.

BACTERIAL VAGINOSIS

The organisms most commonly associated with bacterial vaginosis (BV) are
- *Gardnerella vaginalis* (most abundant),
- Bacteroides,
- Mobiluncus spp.
- *Mycoplasma hominis*.

The principal symptom is the occurrence of an offensive, fishy smelling, yellowish discharge, without pruritus. Trichomonas infection also causes a similar discharge but with pruritus.

However, it can be symptomless in many women.

Diagnosis

- Presence of clue cells on microscopic examination of a saline smear is the most specific criterion for diagnosing bacterial vaginosis. Clue cells are vaginal epithelial cells with bacteria adherent to their surfaces. The edges of the squamous epithelial cells become studded with bacteria. (The epithelial cells appear to be peppered with coccobacilli.)
- Gram stained smear will show predominantly Gardnerella and/or Mobiluncus morphotypes with a few or absent Lactobacilli.

In clinical practice BV can be diagnosed by using the Amsel criteria:
- Thin, white or yellow discharge with a fishy odour.
- Clue cells on microscopy.
- pH of vaginal fluid >4.5.
- Release of a fishy odour on adding 10% potassium hydroxide (KOH).

At least three criteria should be present.

Complications During Pregnancy

- Preterm labour
- Prelabour rupture of membranes
- Chorioamnionitis

Treatment

- **Oral metronidazole** 400 mg administered twice a day for 7 days is the most effective treatment. A single dose of 2 gm may result in recurrence. Consumption of alcohol should be avoided for at least 48 hours after the treatment as metronidazole reacts with alcohol.
- One full applicator (5 gm) of metronidazole gel 0.75% is inserted into the vagina daily for 5 days.
- **Clindamycin** cream 2%, one full applicator (5 gm) intravaginally at bedtime for 7 days.
- **Oral clindamycin** 300 mg is given twice daily for 7 days.

TRICHOMONIASIS

It is a sexually transmitted infection, caused by *Trichomonas vaginalis* which is a motile protozoa.

Symptoms

- Vulvovaginitis with a purulent, offensive, greenish yellow, frothy, vaginal discharge.
- Pruritus is a characteristic symptom.

Diagnosis

- A clinical diagnosis is made by the history of pruritus and by observing the characteristic discharge.
- Microscopy of vaginal secretions mixed with saline will demonstrate the motile organism, which is identified from its shape and four moving flagellae.
- The diagnosis can be further confirmed by culture, in the Feinberg-Whittington medium.
- The patient and the partner should be tested for other sexually transmitted infections.

Treatment

- Metronidazole, either 2 gm as a single dose, or 400 mg twice a day for 5 days.
- The partner should be treated before resuming intercourse together.

Trichomonas and Candida are the only infections which cause pruritus.

CHLAMYDIA

Many infections are asymptomatic, or there can be a white mucoid discharge resembling the physiological discharge.

Chlamydia Causes

- cervicitis,
- pelvic inflammatory disease,
- trachoma,
- conjunctivitis,
- lymphogranuloma venereum,
- proctitis.

The infectious particles are the elementary bodies that infect columnar epithelial cells.

Diagnosis

- It is essential that samples are collected from the endocervix and areas of cervical ectropion, so that columnar epithelial cells are harvested.
- The following tests can be performed.
  - Nucleic acid amplification tests such as the PCR are very sensitive and can be performed on urine or endocervical swabs.
  - Enzyme linked immunosorbent assay (ELISA) tests can be performed on endocervical swabs, but their sensitivity is limited.
  - Direct fluorescent antibody tests.
  - Culture of the organism.
- The PCR test is the most reliable test. It is non-invasive and can be used for screening.
- The woman and her partner must be tested for other sexually transmitted infections.

Treatment

The following drugs are effective and both partners should be treated.

- Doxycycline 100 mg administered twice daily for 7 days. This is the treatment of choice.
- A single dose of azithromycin 1 gm.
- Ofloxacin 400 mg administered daily for 7 days.

Pregnant women are treated with one of the following drugs:

- A single dose of azithromycin 1 gm.
- Erythromycin 500 mg administered twice daily for 14 days.

GONORRHOEA

Neisseria gonorrhoeae is an intracellular gram-negative diplococcus, which colonizes columnar or cuboidal epithelium. It does not colonise the stratified squamous epithelium which covers the vagina.

Symptoms

- Cervicitis with purulent discharge.
- Urethritis with dysuria and purulent discharge.
- Proctitis.
- Conjunctivitis in the newborn.
- Upper genital tract infection.

The woman may complaint of purulent vaginal discharge, dysuria, and lower abdominal pain or may be symptomless. Examination may be normal or may reveal lower abdominal tenderness, cervicitis with mucopurulent discharge or adnexal tenderness.

Diagnosis

- Gram-stained smears of cervical or urethral swabs are examined for gram-negative intracellular diplococci. It is less reliable in women but is sensitive in urethral swabs in men.
- DNA amplification tests (PCR) are reliable and sensitive and are performed on material obtained from endocervical swabs.
- The organism can be cultured in a medium of blood agar and antibiotics (to inhibit the growth of other organisms) in the presence of a carbon dioxide concentration of 7%. It is sensitive and can be combined with an antibiotic sensitivity test.
- The woman and the partner should be screened for other sexually transmitted infections.

Treatment

The following drugs are effective
- A single dose of oral amoxycillin 1 gm with probenecid 2 gm as a single dose.
- A single dose of oral ciprofloxacin 500 mg
- A single intramuscular injection of spectinomycin 2 gm.
- A single dose of oral azithromycin 1 gm.
- A single intramuscular injection of ceftriaxone 250 mg.
- A single dose of oral cefixime 400 mg.
- However, *N. gonorrhoea* has developed resistance to many antimicrobials. Therefore, following combined regimes containing a cephalosporin is recommended as effective treatment regimes.
  - Ceftriaxone 250 mg IM in a single dose plus azithromycin 1 gm orally as a single dose or oral cefixime 400 mg as a single dose plus azithromycin 1 gm orally as a single dose. This regime has the advantage of being effective against Chlamydia as well, as it contains azithromycin.
- Both partners should be treated.
- They should refrain from sex till the treatment is complete.

PELVIC INFLAMMATORY DISEASE (PID)

PID is the result of infection ascending from the endocervix causing:
- endometritis,
- salpingitis,
- parametritis,
- oophoritis,
- tubo-ovarian abscess,
- pelvic peritonitis.

Causative Organisms

- *Neisseria gonorrhoeae* and *Chlamydia trachomatis* account for more than 25% of cases.
- *Gardnerella vaginalis*.
- Anaerobes.
- *Mycoplasma genitalium*.

Symptoms

- Fever in acute cases
- Bilateral lower abdominal pain.
- Deep dyspareunia.
- Purulent offensive vaginal discharge.
- Secondary dysmenorrhea, intermenstrual bleeding and heavy menstrual bleeding.

Signs

- High temperature (more than 38°C) in the acute stage.
- Bilateral lower abdominal tenderness.
- Presence of cervicitis on speculum examination
- Cervical motion tenderness on bimanual vaginal examination.
- Adnexal tenderness on bimanual vaginal examination. Presence of a tender adnexal mass.

Diagnosis

- Diagnosis is difficult as symptoms and signs are most often non-specific. It may be symptomatic or asymptomatic.
- It is a clinical diagnosis based on history, signs and symptoms.
- ESR, C-reactive protein and the white cell count may be elevated in acute cases but is non-specific and may not be always present in chronic cases.
- Test for Chlamydia and gonorrhoea. A positive result supports the diagnosis.
- Endocervical swab for microscopy and culture. The absence of pus cells in material obtained from the endocervix or the vagina has a negative predictive value (95%) in the diagnosis of PID but their presence is not regarded as specific.
- Ultrasound scan to exclude a tubo-ovarian mass or a pelvic abscess.
- Laparoscopy may be done to detect an adnexal mass and adhesions in chronic cases, but is not indicated to diagnose acute cases.

Differential Diagnosis

- Ectopic pregnancy
  - Should be excluded in all women suspected of having acute PID.
- Acute appendicitis
  - Nausea and vomiting occur in appendicitis, but only in 50% of those with acute PID. Cervical movement pain is less common in appendicitis.
- Endometriosis
  - Both endometriosis and chronic pelvic infections cause chronic pelvic pain, dysmenorrhoea, dyspareunia, short menstrual cycles and infertility.
- Torsion or rupture of an ovarian cyst
  - Often of sudden onset and a cyst may detected on examination or on ultrasound scanning
- Urinary tract infection
  - The patient may present with dysuria and/or frequency.
- Functional pain
  - May be associated with long-standing symptoms and can mimic chronic PID.

Management

- Outpatient treatment is possible in mild to moderate cases.
- Admission is needed in more serious patients needing intravenous therapy and/or surgery for pelvic abscess or peritonitis.
- Treatment should be commenced early in suspected cases to prevent long-term sequelae.
- Rest and analgesics are required, especially in the acute phase.
- Intravenous fluids and antibiotics are necessary in acute cases.

Antibiotic Treatment

- Is directed towards Chlamydia, gonorrhoea and anaerobic organisms.
- A single intramuscular injection of ceftriaxone 500 mg together with oral doxycycline 100 mg twice daily and metronidazole 400 mg twice daily for 14 days. This is the treatment of choice as it covers gonococcus, Chlamydia and anaerobes.
- Oral ofloxacin 400 mg twice daily and oral metronidazole 400 mg twice daily for 14 days. (Not recommended in gonococcal infections due to increased resistance to these drugs.)
- Levofloxacin 500 mg once daily for 14 days could be used as an alternative to ofloxacin.
- Metronidazole is included to improve coverage for anaerobic bacteria.

Surgery

Laparoscopy is indicated for adhesiolysis in chronic cases.

Treatment of the Sexual Partners

The woman and her partner should be tested for gonococcus, Chlamydia, HIV and other sexually transmitted infections.

The man should be given appropriate antibiotics.

They should avoid unprotected sexual intercourse till the treatment is completed.

SEXUALLY TRANSMITTED INFECTIONS

- Are caused by more than 30 different bacteria, viruses and parasites.
- Common bacterial and parasitic infections are syphilis, gonorrhoea, Chlamydia (including lymphogranuloma venereum), bacterial vaginosis and trichomoniasis.
- Less common bacterial infections are chancroid caused by *Haemophilus ducreyi* and granuloma inguinale caused by *Klebsiella granulomatis*.
- These infections can be cured by antimicrobial therapy.
- Common viral infections are hepatitis B, HIV, herpes simplex virus and human papillomavirus infections. These are not curable, but the infections can be modified or reduced by early treatment.
- Sexually transmitted infections are spread predominantly through sexual contact.

- Syphilis, hepatitis B and HIV are also spread through blood and blood products.
- Chlamydia, gonorrhea, hepatitis B, HIV, genital herpes and syphilis can be transmitted from mother to child during pregnancy and childbirth.

Diagnosis

- **Syphilis**
  - VDRL test is the first screening test.
  - If it is positive, the diagnosis should be confirmed by performing a specific test, such as fluorescent treponemal antibody test or *Treponema pallidum* haemagglutination test.
- **Genital herpes**
  - Electron microscopy of material obtained from the ulcers
- **HIV and hepatitis B**
  - Diagnosed by specific blood tests.
- **Chancroid**
  - Diagnosed by clinical features.
  - The organism may be cultured from the material obtained from an ulcer.
- **Granuloma inguinale**
  - Demonstration of Donovan bodies in a biopsy from the lesion.

Treatment

- Lymphogranuloma venereum
  - Doxycycline, 100 mg orally, twice daily for 14 days or oral erythromycin, 500 mg 4 times daily for 14 days.

- Syphilis
  - A single intramuscular injection of 2.4 million IU benzathine benzylpenicillin is very effective. Because of the volume involved, this dose is usually given as two injections at separate sites.
  - Intramuscular injection of 1.2 million IU of procaine benzylpenicillin, daily for 10 consecutive days.
  - Penicillin-allergic non-pregnant patients can be given doxycycline, 100 mg orally, twice daily for 14 days, while pregnant patients are given erythromycin, 500 mg orally, 4 times daily for 14 days.
- Chancroid
  - Oral ciprofloxacin, 500 mg twice daily for 3 days.
  - Erythromycin 500 mg orally, 4 times daily for 7 days.
  - Oral azithromycin, 1 gm as a single dose.
- Granuloma inguinale
  - Azithromycin, 1 gm orally on first day followed by 500 mg orally, once a day.
  - Doxycycline, 100 mg orally, twice daily
  - The treatment regime should be continued until all lesions have completely healed.
- Genital warts
  - Local application of podophyllin.
  - Diathermy cauterisation.
- Genital herpes
  - Acyclovir 200 mg 5 times a day for 7 days.

QUESTIONS

1. **A woman complains of clear mucoid, non-offensive vaginal discharge without pruritus or soreness. She is infertile due to a tubal factor. The cervix appears inflamed on speculum examination.**

   What is the most likely cause of her symptoms?

   A. Bacterial vaginosis.
   B. Chlamydial infection.

   C. Gonorrhoea.
   D. Leucorrhoea.
   E. Tricomoniasis.

2. **A woman complains of clear mucoid, non-offensive vaginal discharge without pruritus or soreness. The cervix appears inflamed on speculum examination and an endocervical swab is taken.**
   What is the most appropriate test to confirm the diagnosis?

A. Perform electron microscopic examination.

B. Perform a culture.

C. Perform a direct fluorescent antibody test.

D. Perform a DNA amplification (PCR) test.

E. Perform an ELISA test.

3. **A woman, who is on oral contraceptive pills, presents with a whitish vaginal discharge. She does not have soreness or itching. The discharge causes yellowish stains in her underwear. pH of the discharge is acidic. Microscopy shows normal numbers of lactobacilli.**

   Which one of the following is the most appropriate diagnosis?

   A. Bacterial vaginosis.

   B. Cervical polyp.

   C. Chlamydial infection.

   D. Leucorrhoea.

   E. Vaginal candidiasis.

4. **A multiparous woman complains of an offensive fishy smelling yellowish discharge without pruritus. Her previous pregnancy had ended in a preterm delivery.**

   Which of the following is the best test to confirm the diagnosis?

   A. Culture the vaginal discharge.

   B. Microscopic examination of a gram-stained smear of the vaginal discharge.

   C. Microscopic examination of a wet mount of the vaginal discharge.

   D. Perform a white cell count.

   E. Test the vaginal pH.

5. **A woman complains of an offensive, fishy smelling and yellowish vaginal discharge with pruritus.**

   Which of the following is the best test to confirm the diagnosis?

A. Culture the vaginal discharge.

B. Direct microscopic examination of the vaginal discharge mixed with saline.

C. Microscopic examination of a gram-stained smear of the vaginal discharge.

D. Perform a white cell count.

E. Test the vaginal pH.

6. **A woman complains of an offensive fishy smelling yellowish discharge without pruritus. The vaginal pH is >4.5. Gram-stained vaginal smear shows a reduced number of lactobacilli with a large number of *Gardnerella vaginalis*.**

   What is the most likely cause of her symptoms?

   A. Bacterial Vaginosis.

   B. Chlamydial infection.

   C. Gonorrhoea.

   D. Leucorrhoea.

   E. Trichomoniasis.

7. **A woman complains of an offensive fishy smelling yellowish discharge without pruritus. Vaginal pH is greater than 4.5. Gram-stained vaginal smear shows a reduced number of lactobacilli with a large number of *Gardnerella vaginalis*.**

   What is the best treatment option for this patient?

   A. Clindamycin 300 mg twice daily for 7 days.

   B. Clindamycin vaginal gel once a day for 7 days.

   C. Metronidazole 400 mg twice a day for 7 days.

   D. Metronidazole 2 gm as a single dose.

   E. Metronidazole vaginal gel once a day for 7 days.

8. **A woman complains of purulent vaginal discharge and dysuria. Vaginal examination reveals cervicitis and tenderness in the adnexal region.**

   Which of the following tests is the best to confirm the diagnosis?

A. Endocervical swab for Gram staining.

B. Endocervical swab for nucleic acid amplification tests.

C. High vaginal swab for nucleic acid amplification tests.

D. High vaginal swab for culture and ABST.

E. Perform a white cell count.

9. **A woman presents with a complaint of white mucoid vaginal discharge. PCR testing is performed on material obtained from the endocervix and Chlamydia is identified.**

   Which one of the following drugs cannot be used to treat this patient?

   A. Azithromycin

   B. Doxycycline

   C. Erythromycin

   D. Metronidazole

   E. Ofloxacin

10. **A woman presents to the antenatal clinic with a complaint of white mucoid vaginal discharge at a period of amenorrhoea of 12 weeks. PCR testing is performed on material obtained from the endocervix and Chlamydia is identified.**

    Which one of the following drugs is most suitable to treat this patient?

    A. Amoxycillin

    B. Doxycycline

    C. Erythromycin

    D. Metronidazole

    E. Ofloxacin

11. **A woman complains of purulent vaginal discharge. Vaginal examination reveals cervicitis and tenderness in the adnexal region. Microscopic examination of a gram-stained smear of endocervical discharge reveals the presence of gram-negative intracellular diplococcic.**

    What is the best treatment option?

A. Amoxycillin 1 gm with probenecid 2 gm as a single oral dose,

B. Cefixime 400 mg orally as a single dose and azithromycin 1g orally as a single dose.

C. Ceftriaxone 250 mg IM in a single dose and azithromycin 1g orally as a single dose.

D. Ciprofloxacin 500 mg and azithromycin 1gm as a single oral dose.

E. Spectinomycin 2 gm as a single intramuscular dose.

12. **A 30-year-old multiparous woman complains of a painless ulcer in the vulva. She has several sexual partners. Her previous pregnancy has ended in a stillbirth at 24 weeks.**

    What is the first test which should be performed to arrive at a diagnosis?

    A. Blood test for HIV.

    B. Culture of scraping from the ulcer.

    C. Electron microscopy of scraping from the ulcer.

    D. Nucleic acid amplification tests (PCR) of scraping from the ulcer.

    E. Venereal Disease Research Laboratory (VDRL) test.

13. **A 30-year-old multiparous woman complains of a painless ulcer in the vulva. She has several sexual partners. The VDRL test is positive.**

    What is the next test which should be performed to confirm the diagnosis?

    A. Culture of scraping from the ulcer.

    B. Electron microscopy of scraping from the ulcer.

    C. Enzyme linked immune assay test.

    D. Fluorescent treponemal antibody test.

    E. Nucleic acid amplification test (PCR) of scraping from the ulcer.

14. **A 30-year-old multiparous woman complains of a painless ulcer in the vulva. She has several sexual partners. A diagnosis of syphilis is made.**

    What is the best treatment option?

A. A single dose of Benzathine ben-zylpenicillin, 2.4 million IU by intra-muscular injection.

B. Ceftriaxone 250 mg IM in a single dose and azithromycin 1gm orally as a single dose.

C. Doxycycline, 100 mg orally, twice daily for 14 days.

D. Erythromycin, 500 mg orally, 4 times daily for 14 days.

E. Procaine benzylpenicillin, 1.2 million IU by intramuscular injection, daily for 10 consecutive days.

15. A woman complains of multiple small painful ulcers of the vulva of 2 days duration. She had a previous similar episode which healed spontaneously.

What is the most likely diagnosis?

A. Chancroid
B. Genital herpes
C. Granuloma inguinale
D. Lymphogranuloma venerum
E. Primary syphilis

16. A woman complains of multiple small painful ulcers of the vulva of 2 days duration. She had a previous similar episode which healed spontaneously.

Which of the following is the best test to diagnose the infection?

A. Culture of scraping from the ulcers.
B. Electron microscopy of scraping from the ulcers.

C. Enzyme linked immune assay test.
D. Microscopic examination of a gram-stained smear from the ulcers.
E. Nucleic acid amplification tests (PCR) of scraping from the ulcers.

17. Which of the following infective conditions are not caused by *Chlamydia trachomatis*?

A. Chancroid
B. Conjunctivitis
C. Lymphogranuloma venereum
D. Proctitis
E. Trachoma

18. A 30-year-old woman complains of lower abdominal pain and purulent vaginal discharge. The temperature is 38.5°C and the white cell count and C-reactive protein levels are elevated. She has bilateral lower abdominal tenderness, cervical motion pain and the cervix appears inflamed on speculum examination.

What is the best treatment option?

A. A single IM injection of ceftriaxone 500 mg with oral doxycycline and oral metronidazole for 14 days.
B. Ceftriaxone 250 mg IM in a single dose with oral azithromycin for 14 days.
C. Oral levofloxacin and oral metroni-dazole for 14 days.
D. Oral metronidazole for 14 days.
E. Oral ofloxacin and oral metronidazole for 14 days.

ANSWERS AND EXPLANATIONS

Q. 1 (B)

This woman has clear, mucoid, non-offen-sive, vaginal discharge, cervicitis and tubal damage. Therefore, the likely diagnosis is chlamydial infection. Bacterial vaginosis and trichomoniasis cause yellowish offensive discharge and the latter causes pruritus. Gonorrhoea causes cervicitis and tubal damage but the discharge is purulent. Leucorrhoea causes only a white vaginal discharge.

Q. 2 (D)

This woman most probably has chlamydial infection as she has a white mucoid vaginal discharge without pruritus and cervicitis. DNA amplification tests, such as the PCR are very sensitive for diagnosing

Chlamydia and can be performed on urine or endocervical swabs. This is regarded as the best test to diagnose Chlamydia infection. It is non-invasive and can be used as a screening test. The samples should be collected from the endocervix so that columnar epithelial cells can be harvested, because Chlamydia does not infect stratified squamous epithelium. Enzyme linked immunosorbent assay (ELISA) tests and direct fluorescent antibody tests can be performed on endocervical swabs but their sensitivity is limited. Cultures or microscopy are not necessary to diagnose chlamydial infection.

Q. 3 (D)

This woman has leucorrhoea because she has white vaginal discharge without pruritus or soreness and the normal number of lactobacilli are present. Chlamydia will cause a similar discharge, but the number of lactobacilli will be reduced, as there is an infection. Vaginal candidiasis will cause a similar discharge, but pruritus will be a prominent symptom. A cervical polyp will cause a blood stained or purulent discharge. Bacterial vaginosis will cause a yellowish offensive discharge.

Q. 4 (C)

This woman most probably has bacterial vaginosis, as she has a non-pruritic, offen-sive yellowish discharge and has a past history of preterm labour. Clue cells can be visualised on microscopic examination of a wet mount of the vaginal discharge with a drop of saline. Clue cells are characteristic of bacterial vaginosis. Therefore, the diagnosis can be confirmed as she has two of the Amsel criteria. Gram-stained smear will show predominantly Gardnerella and/or Mobiluncus morphotypes with a few or absent Lactobacilli, but demonstration of clue cells in a wet smear is more specific. The pH should be more than 4.5 and this is included in the Amsel criteria. Culture of

the vaginal discharge or a white cell count is not used in the diagnosis of bacterial vaginosis.

Q. 5 (B)

This woman most probably has tricho-moniasis as she has a fishy smelling, yellowish vaginal discharge with pruritus. Microscopy of vaginal secretions mixed with saline will confirm the diagnosis, by demonstrating the motile organism, which is identified from its shape and four moving flagellae. Culture in the Feinberg-Whittington medium may be necessary to confirm the diagnosis, especially if the direct smear is negative.

Q. 6 (A)

A diagnosis of bacterial vaginosis can be made as she has a yellow, offensive discharge, without pruritus and the vaginal pH is more than 4.5 (two Amsel criteria). Also microscopic examination of a gram-stained smear, which shows reduced numbers of lactobacilli, with G. vaginalis, gram-negative rods and cocci support the diagnosis. Trichomoniasis will cause a similar discharge, but with pruritus as a prominent symptom. Chlamydia will cause a white discharge. Leucorrhoea will cause a white discharge and the lactobacilli will not be reduced. Gonorrhoea will cause a purulent discharge and the woman will have vaginal soreness and/or dysuria. A gram-stained smear will show gram-negative intracellular diplococci.

Q. 7 (C)

This woman has bacterial vaginosis. The best treatment option is oral metronidazole 400 mg twice daily for 7 days. However, the other treatment options are also effective.

Q. 8 (B)

This woman most probably has gonococcal infection, as she has a purulent vaginal discharge with dysuria, cervicitis and adnexal tenderness. Examination of gram-stained smears of endocervical or urethral swabs for gram-negative intracellular diplococcic is less reliable in women, but is sensitive in urethral swabs in men. Nucleic acid amplification tests such as PCR are sensitive, when performed on endocervical swabs and is regarded as the most appropriate diagnostic test for gonorrhoea. The organism does not infect stratified squamous epithelium and cannot be detected in a high vaginal swab. The organism can be cultured in a medium of blood agar and antibiotics (to inhibit the growth of other organisms) in the presence of a carbon dioxide concentration of 7 per cent. This can be combined with an antibiotic sensitivity test.

Q. 9 (D)

Of the above drugs only metronidazole cannot be used to treat Chlamydia.

Q. 10 (C)

Only erythromycin and azithromycin can be used to treat pregnant women with chlamydial infection.

Q. 11 (C)

This patient has gonorrhoea and the best treatment option is a single intramuscular injection of ceftriaxone 250 mg IM and a single oral dose of azithromycin 1 gm. Azithromycin is effective against Chlamydia as well. However, ceftriaxone is also effective against Chlamydia. If ceftriaxone is not available or if the patient refuses intramuscular injection, a single oral dose of cefixime 400 mg with a single oral dose of azithromycin 1 g, is an equally effective regime against gonorrhoea and Chlamydia.

Q. 12 (E)

Q. 13 (D)

Q. 14 (A)

Explanation for questions 12, 13, 14

The most probable diagnosis is primary syphilis for the following reasons:

- She has a single painless ulcer
- She has multiple sexual partners
- She has had a mid-trimester stillbirth

Therefore, the VDRL test which is the initial screening test for syphilis should be performed first. Culture of scrapings from the ulcer is done to confirm chancroid, while electron microscopy is done to confirm genital herpes. Nucleic acid amplification test is done to confirm Chlamydia and gonorrhoea. Enzyme linked immune assay test can be done to diagnose Chlamydia and lymphogranuloma venereum.

The VDRL test is a non-specific test which can be positive in autoimmune conditions. Therefore, if the VDRL test is positive, a specific treponemal test, such as the *Treponema pallidum* haemagglutination test, or the fluorescent treponemal antibody test, should be done to confirm the diagnosis. The latter is the most sensitive test, though time consuming to perform.

Once the diagnosis of syphilis is confirmed, the best treatment option is a single intramuscular injection of benzathine benzylpenicillin, 2.4 million IU. It is effective and eliminates the problem of default by the patient, unlike treatment with procaine penicillin which though effective has to be given for 10 days. Penicillin-allergic non-pregnant patients can be given doxycycline, 100 mg orally, twice daily for 14 days, while pregnant patients are given erythromycin, 500 mg orally, 4 times daily for 14 days. Ceftriaxone is given for gonococcal infections.

Q. 15 (B)

The diagnosis is genital herpes because she has multiple small painful ulcers and a history of a previous similar episode which could be the primary infection. Chancroid also can cause similar painful ulcers, but these last for a long time and cause lymph node enlargement. Lymphogranuloma venereum causes a small shallow ulcer with lymph node enlargement. Granuloma inguinale causes papules and ulcers with lymphedema. Primary syphilis causes a single painless ulcer.

Q. 16 (B)

Electron microscopy of scrapings from ulcers is done to confirm genital herpes, while culture is done to confirm chancroid. Nucleic acid amplification test is done to confirm Chlamydia and gonorrhoea. Enzyme linked immune assay test can be done to diagnose Chlamydia and lymphogranuloma venerum. Microscopic examination of a gram-stained smear is done to demonstrate gonococcus.

Q. 17 (A)

Chlamydia causes cervicitis, pelvic inflammatory disease, trachoma, conjunctivitis, lymphogranuloma venereum, and proctitis. Chancroid is caused by *Haemophilus ducreyi*.

Q. 18 (A)

Acute pelvic inflammatory disease is a clinical diagnosis. A diagnosis of acute PID can be made in this young woman as she has lower abdominal pain, fever, purulent vaginal discharge together with lower abdominal tenderness and cervicitis. This is further confirmed by the high white cell count and C-reactive protein levels. Ultrasound scan is performed if a pelvic abscess is suspected. Laparoscopy is not essential to diagnose acute PID.

Once the diagnosis is made the treatment schedule should include antibiotics which are effective against Chlamydia, gonorrhoea and anaerobic organisms. Therefore, the best treatment option is a combination of ceftriaxone (which is highly effective against gonorrhoea), doxycycline (which is effective against Chlamydia) and metronidazole which is effective against anaerobes.

REFERENCE

- UK National Guideline for the Management of Pelvic Inflammatory Disease 2011 (updated June 2011).

10

Infertility

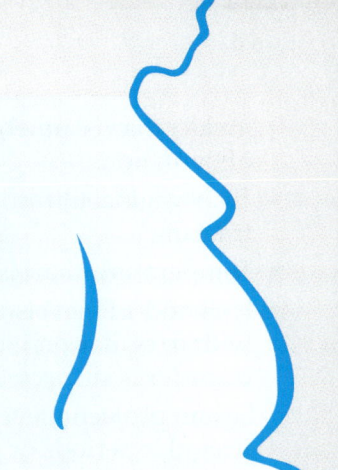

A woman of reproductive age, who has not conceived after 1 year of unprotected vaginal sexual intercourse, in the absence of any known cause of infertility, should be offered further clinical assessment and investigations along with her partner.

Offer an earlier referral for specialist consultation if:

- – the woman is aged 36 years or older,
- – there is a known clinical cause of infertility or a history of predisposing factors for infertility.
- Women who are trying to conceive should have regular sexual intercourse once in 2 days.
- BMI of over 30 and below 19 are associated with reduced fertility.
- Avoid smoking, alcohol, caffeinated beverages and unprescribed drugs.
- Men should avoid tight underwear and exposure to heat.

History from the woman should include:
- previous pregnancies/miscarriages,
- contraceptive use,
- frequency of sexual intercourse and problems associated with intercourse,
- regular periods, dysmenorrhea,
- history of sexually transmitted disease/pelvic inflammatory disease/endometriosis, endocrine disorders, chronic illnesses

such as diabetes and tuberculosis. History of previous surgeries,
- use of prescribed and unprescribed drugs, exposure to irradiation and toxins,
- previous investigations and previous treatment.

History from the male partner should include:
- previous history of fathering a child,
- use of prescribed and unprescribed drugs,
- problems associated with intercourse,
- history of mumps, orchitis, chronic illnesses and surgeries,
- exposure to heat, radiation and toxins,
- smoking and alcohol,
- previous investigations and previous treatment.

INVESTIGATIONS

- The first step is to perform a seminal fluid analysis because,
  - – it is a non-invasive, easy investigation.
  - – male infertility is common.

Tests for Ovulation

- The best test is the day 21 progesterone level, because it is a non-invasive easy test, which can be repeated. Even women having regular cycles should be offered this test. If the cycle is longer than 28 days, the test has to be performed at a later day. A value greater than 30 nmol/L indicates occurrence of ovulation.

- Transvaginal ultrasound scans for follicular tracking.
- Temperature chart is not recommended.
- FSH and LH levels are done only in those with irregular periods where an ovulatory disorder is suspected.
- Serum prolactin levels are done if there are irregular periods or galactorrhoea.
- Thyroid function tests should be done only in women with symptoms of thyroid disease.
- Endometrial biopsy to evaluate the luteal phase is of no value as medical treatment of luteal phase defects do not improve pregnancy rates.

Parameters Used to Test for Ovarian Reserve

A good response to gonadotropin stimulation occurs if,
- patient's age is less than 40 years
- the total antral count is more than 16
- the anti-müllerian hormone level is more than 25 pmol/L
- FSH is less than 4 IU/L

Tests for Tubal Patency

- Hysterosalpingography
  - It is a reliable test for tubal patency and it is less invasive and makes more efficient use of resources than laparoscopy.
  - It is offered to women who are not known to have co-morbidities, such as pelvic inflammatory disease, previous ectopic pregnancy or endometriosis.
- Laparoscopy
  - It is the appropriate test for tubal patency if other pelvic pathologies are present, as these can be diagnosed and treated at the same time.

Women undergoing treatment should be tested for rubella status, HIV, hepatitis B and Chlamydia. Folic acid should be commenced.

TREATMENT

Suspected Ovulatory Disorders

WHO group 1 ovulatory disorders (hypothalamic amenorrhoea or hypogonadotropic hypogonadism)
- Increase body weight if the BMI is less than 19.
- Reduce exercise.
- Pulsatile administration of gonadotropin-releasing hormone or gonadotropins to induce ovulation.
  - Administer FSH 75 IU intramuscularly daily from the second day of the period and hCG 5000 IU intramuscularly when the follicle reaches 1.8 cm.
  - Administration of GnRH in a pulsatile fashion by means of a computerized infusion pump, either subcutaneously 5 to 20 mcg every 90 minutes or intravenously 25 mcg every 90 minutes can induce ovulation in anovulatory conditions, such as hypothalamic amenorrhea and polycystic ovarian disease.

WHO group 2 ovulatory disorders
- Reduce weight if the BMI is > than 30.
- Treat with metformin.
- Induce ovulation.
  - Clomiphene citrate is the usual first line drug. 50–100 mg daily is given for 5 days from the second day of menstruation. It can be combined with metformin especially in obese women.
  - Letrazole 5 mg daily, for five days from the second day of the period, can be used to induce ovulation in those with PCOS.
  - Maximum duration of treatment is 6 cycles.
  - TVS should be done for follicular tracking and to exclude hyperstimulation.
  - Treatment can be combined with injection of 5000 IU of hCG when the pre-ovulatory follicle reaches 1.8–2 cm.

- Second line therapy for those not responding to clomiphene
  - Treatment with gonadotropins
  - Laparoscopic ovarian drilling is done for women with PCOS who are resistant to ovulation induction alone.
- Women with hyperprolactinaemia may need intracranial investigations. Treatment is with dopamine agonists such as bromocriptine or cabergoline in the absence of a pituitary macroadenoma.

Tubal Disorders
  - Tubal surgery
  - Assisted reproduction

MALE INFERTILITY

The first step in investigating an infertile couple is to perform a seminal fluid analysis.

Normal Seminal Fluid Analysis
- Volume: 2 ml or more
- Liquefaction time: Within 60 minutes
- pH: 7.2 or more
- Sperm concentration: 15 million spermatozoa per ml or more
- Total sperm number: 39 million spermatozoa per ejaculate or more
- Motility: 40% or more motile (grades a and b) or 32% or more with progressive motility (grade a) within 60 minutes of ejaculation
- Vitality: 58% or more live
- White blood cells: Fewer than 1 million per ml
- Morphology: >4% normal forms

Method of Collection
- Abstain for 2–3 days.
- Collect the specimen into a sterile wide mouthed plastic pot by masturbation.
- Take the specimen to the lab as soon as possible. It is better to collect the specimen in the laboratory premises.

Abnormalities
- Oligozoospermia (<15 million spermatozoa/ml)
- Asthenozoospermia (<40% motile spermatozoa)
- Teratozoospermia (<4% normal forms).

Quite often, all three pathologies occur at the same time, i.e. as oligo-asthenoteratozoospermia (OAT) syndrome.

If any abnormality is found, a repeat test is ideally performed in 3 months, to allow a complete cycle of spermatogenesis to take place.

Causes
Abnormalities may be due to:
- hypothalamic pituitary failure: Hypogonadotropic hypogonadism,
- primary testicular failure: Hypergonadotropic hypogonadism,
- obstruction of the genital tract.
- hyperprolactinaemia, thyroid and other endocrine abnormalities

Causes of Hypogonadotropic Hypogonadism (Hypothalamic/Pituitary Failure with Low FSH and LH)
- Congenital anomalies—isolated hypogonadotropic hypogonadism (IHH), Kallmann's syndrome.
- Acquired anomalies—acquired hypothalamic/pituitary gland diseases (tumours hyperprolactinaemia, granulomatous illness, hemochromatosis)
- Exogenous factors—drugs (anabolic steroids), obesity, head injuries, irradiation.

Causes of Hypergonadotropic Hypogonadism—Testicular Failure (High FSH and LH)
- Congenital—Klinefelter's syndrome (XXY), anorchia, cryptorchidism, testicular dysgenesis, Y chromosome microdeletions.
- Acquired—orchitis, testicular torsion, testicular tumour, systemic illness, cytotoxic therapy, radiation.

FURTHER INVESTIGATIONS

Serum FSH, LH, Prolactin, Testosterone and Thyroid Hormone Levels

- These hormone levels will help to differentiate between obstructive and non-obstructive causes.
- If the hormone levels are normal and the testicular volume is normal, the azoospermia is due to an obstructive cause.
- If FSH, LH and testosterone levels are low, the failure is due to a hypothalamic or pituitary cause, or due to use of anabolic steroids. CT/MRI scan of the pituitary may be needed.
- If FSH and LH levels are high and the testicular volume is reduced, primary testicular failure is present.

Genetic Evaluation and Karyotyping

- These are needed if congenital causes of testicular failure are suspected.

Microbiological Testing

Microscopy and culture is needed if there are more than 1 million pus cells.

Testicular Biopsy

Biopsy is done if the testicular volume and FSH are normal, to differentiate between testicular insufficiency and obstruction of the male genital tract.

TREATMENT

Counselling

- Lifestyle factors can impair semen quality.
- Should stop heavy smoking, alcohol abuse, use of anabolic steroids and extreme sports (marathon training, excessive strength sports).
- Should prevent an increase in scrotal temperature through thermal underwear, sauna, hot tub use, or occupational exposure to heat sources.
- A considerable number of drugs can affect spermatogenesis.

Hormone Treatment can be Tried in those with Hypogonadotropic Hypogonadism

- Clomiphene citrate 50 mg/day or tamoxifen 20 mg/day.
- In those not responding to treatment commence hCG injections 1500 IU three times a week. If the response is poor, add HMG or FSH 75–150 IU intramuscularly 3 times per week, until adequate spermatogenesis occurs.
- Bromocriptine is used to treat hyperprolactinaemia.
- Other hormonal disorders should be treated.

Surgical Treatment

- Microsurgery/vasovasostomy and epididymovasostomy for obstructive causes. If not successful carry out aspiration of sperms and intracytoplasmic sperm injection.
- The value of treating a varicocele is not established.

Treatment of Ejaculatory Failure

- Use of drugs
- Testicular sperm extraction (TESE)

Other Treatment Options

Intrauterine insemination with prepared sperms is recommended in mild non-obstructive abnormalities (if the sperm concentration is more than 5 million/ml).

Donor insemination can be tried for non-obstructive azoospermia.

Testicular sperm extraction is carried out in patients with obstructive azoospermia.

Intracytoplasmic sperm injection and IVF are options for treating male infertility.

QUESTIONS

1. **The best test to determine occurrence of ovulation is:**

   A. Alteration in the consistency of the cervical mucus.

   B. Biphasic changes in the temperature chart.

   C. Detection of a rise in the plasma LH level at mid-cycle.

   D. Elevation of the plasma progesterone levels in the mid-luteal phase.

   E. Occurrence of a plasma oestradiol peak at mid-cycle.

2. **A seminal fluid analysis is performed on the male partner during routine investigation of a couple who have been infertile for 1 year.**

   Which one of the following values could be the cause of their infertility?

   A. 10% progressive motility.

   B. An ejaculatory volume of 3 ml.

   C. Presence 3–4 white blood cells per millilitre.

   D. Presence of 10% normal forms.

   E. Sperm concentration of 30 million/ml.

3. **A man is found to have a sperm concentration of 2 million/ml on one occasion.**

   What is the next step in the management?

   A. Estimate serum FSH and testosterone levels.

   B. Perform testicular aspiration.

   C. Repeat the test in three months.

   D. Repeat the test in three weeks.

   E. Test for antisperm antibodies.

4. **A man is found to have azoospermia on two separate occasions three months apart.**

   What is the next step in the management?

   A. Estimate serum FSH and LH levels.

   B. Perform karyotyping.

   C. Perform a testicular biopsy.

   D. Perform testicular aspiration.

   E. Test for antisperm antibodies.

5. **A man is found to have a sperm concentration of 2 million/ml on two separate occasions three months apart. Serum FSH and LH levels are in the low normal range. MRI scan of the pituitary fossa is normal. The woman has 28-day regular cycles. Investigations reveal regular ovulation and patent tubes.**

   What is the next step in the management?

   A. Advise *in vitro* fertilisation.

   B. Perform artificial insemination with aspirated sperms.

   C. Perform artificial insemination with donor semen.

   D. Treat with clomiphene citrate.

   E. Treat with human chorionic gonadotropin injections.

6. **A man is found to have a sperm concentration of 2 million/ml. Serum FSH and LH levels are low. MRI scan of the pituitary fossa is normal. The sperm concentration improves to 4 million/ml after treatment with clomiphene citrate for 3 months. The woman has 28-day regular cycles. Investigations reveal regular ovulation and patent tubes.**

   What is the most appropriate next step in the management?

   A. Advise *in vitro* fertilisation.

   B. Perform artificial insemination with prepared sperms.

   C. Perform artificial insemination with donor semen.

   D. Treat with hCG followed by FSH injections.

   E. Treat with tamoxifen.

7. **The male partner of an infertile couple has a sperm concentration of 10 million/ml on two separate occasions three months apart. The woman has 28-day regular**

cycles. Investigations reveal regular ovulation and patent tubes.

What is the next step in the management?

A. Artificial insemination after preparation of semen.

B. Artificial insemination with donor semen.

C. Artificial insemination with sperms aspirated from the testes.

D. Treat with clomiphene citrate.

E. Treat with gonadotropin injections.

8. **An infertile woman has menstruation once in 45–60 days. Her BMI is 22. Serum FSH and LH levels are in the low normal range. Mid-luteal progesterone level is 8 nmols/L. Laparoscopy reveals a normal pelvis with patent tubes.**

   What is the first step in the management?

   A. Perform follicular tracking to determine the time of ovulation.

   B. Treat with clomiphene citrate and metformin.

   C. Treat with clomiphene citrate and mid-cycle hCG injections.

   D. Treat with letrozole.

   E. Treat with progestogen in the second half of the cycle.

9. **An infertile woman has menstruation once in 45–60 days. Her BMI is 22. Serum FSH and LH levels are in the low normal range. Serum progesterone level is 8 nmols/L. Laparoscopy reveals a normal pelvis with patent tubes. She was treated with clomiphene citrate for 3 months without success.**

   What is the next step in the management?

   A. *In vitro* fertilisation.

   B. Laparoscopic ovarian drilling.

   C. Treat with clomiphene citrate and metformin.

   D. Treat with FSH injections.

   E. Treat with progestogen in the second half of the cycle.

9a. **An infertile woman has menstruation once in 45–60 days. Her BMI is 22. Serum FSH and LH levels are in the low normal range. Serum progesterone level is 8 nmols/L. Laparoscopy reveals a normal pelvis with patent tubes. She was treated with clomiphene citrate followed by FSH injections without success.**

   What is the next step in the management?

   A. *In vitro* fertilisation.

   B. Laparoscopic ovarian drilling.

   C. Pulsatile administration of GnRH.

   D. Treat with GnRH injections once a month for three months.

   E. Treat with progestogen in the second half of the cycle.

10. **A 30-year-old infertile woman has menstruation once in 45–60 days. Her BMI is 30. Transvaginal ultrasound scan reveals polycystic ovaries. She was advised weight reduction and treated with clomiphene for 3 months without success.**

   What is the next step in the management?

   A. *In vitro* fertilisation.

   B. Laparoscopic ovarian drilling.

   C. Pulsatile administration of gonadotropin releasing hormones.

   D. Treatment with clomiphene and metformin.

   E. Treatment with progestogen in the second half of the cycle.

10a. **A 30-year-old infertile woman has menstruation once in 45–60 days. Her BMI is 30. Transvaginal ultrasound scan reveals polycystic ovaries. She was treated with clomiphene and metformin for 3 months without success.**

   What is the next step in the management?

   A. *In vitro* fertilisation.

   B. Laparoscopic ovarian drilling.

   C. Pulsatile administration of gonadotropin releasing hormones.

   D. Treatment with FSH injections.

   E. Treatment with progestogen in the second half of the cycle.

11. A woman who has been infertile for 2 years attends the clinic. She has regular periods with dysmenorrhoea which is worst on the third day. Laparoscopy reveals peritubal adhesions, patent tubes and pelvic endometriotic deposits.

    What is the next step in the management?

    A. Perform *in vitro* fertilisation.

    B. Perform gamete intrafallopian transfer.

    C. Perform intrauterine insemination.

    D. Perform tubal reconstruction.

    E. Perform adhesiolysis and diathermy cauterisation of the endometriotic deposits.

12. A couple who have failed to conceive after 2 years of unprotected regular intercourse attend the infertility clinic. The woman has 28-day regular periods. They have no other complaints.

    What is the first step in the investigation of this couple?

    A. Maintain a temperature chart.

    B. Perform day 21 progesterone test.

    C. Perform laparoscopy.

    D. Perform seminal fluid analysis.

    E. Perform transvaginal ultrasound scan.

13. A couple who have failed to conceive after 2 years of unprotected regular intercourse attend the infertility clinic. The woman has 28-day regular periods. They have no other complaints. The seminal fluid analysis is normal.

    What is the next step in the investigation of this couple?

    A. Maintain a temperature chart.

    B. Perform a hysterosalpingogram.

    C. Perform a laparoscopy.

    D. Perform day 21 progesterone test.

    E. Perform a transvaginal ultrasound scan for follicular tracking.

14. A 26-year-old woman who has been infertile for 2 years attends the clinic. She has 28-day regular menstrual cycles. Day 21 progesterone level is 30 nmol/L. The seminal fluid analysis is normal. She has no other complaints.

    Which of the following investigations should be performed next?

    A. Hydrotubation.

    B. Hysterosalpingogram.

    C. Laparoscopy and dye test.

    D. Transvaginal ultrasound scanning for follicular tracking.

    E. Tubal insufflation.

15. A 26-year-old woman who has been infertile for 2 years attends the clinic. She has frequent periods with dysmenorrhoea which is worst on the third day. She also complains of deep dyspareunia. Day 21 progesterone level is 30 nmol/L. The seminal fluid analysis is normal.

    Which of the following investigations should be performed next?

    A. Hysterosalpingogram.

    B. Hysteroscopy.

    C. Laparoscopy and dye test.

    D. Transvaginal ultrasound scan for follicular tracking.

    E. Tubal insufflation.

16. Which of the following time periods in the menstrual cycle is most suitable to perform a hysterosalpingogram?

    A. Days 14–21

    B. Days 21–28

    C. Days 3–10

    D. Days 7–11

    E. Days 11–13

ANSWERS AND EXPLANATIONS

Q. 1 (D)

Elevation of the plasma progesterone levels in the luteal phase is the best test for ovulation, because it is non-invasive and a single test performed on the 21st day of a 28-day cycle can confirm ovulation. A value greater than 30 nmol/L indicates occurrence of ovulation. The test will have to be done on about the 28th day in a woman with a longer cycle and may have to be repeated weekly, till a positive value is reached. Transvaginal ultrasound scan to estimate the size of the dominant follicle is a good method to detect ovulation, but several scans may be necessary and it is time consuming. It is used to detect a pre-ovulatory follicle (1.8–2 cm), prior to injection of gonadotropin at mid-cycle, during treatment for ovulation induction. A rise in plasma LH level at the mid-cycle can be used to confirm the time of ovulation, but as the peak is transient, correct timing of the test is difficult. Cervical mucus becomes thinner and can be drawn out into threads at the time of ovulation. Temperature chart depends on the accuracy of testing, as the rise is very small and is hence not an accurate method.

Q. 2 (A)

All the other values except for sperm motility are within the normal range. The normal progressive motility should be more than 32%.

Q. 3 (C)

Q. 4 (A)

Explanation for questions 3 and 4

If an abnormal seminal fluid analysis/low sperm count is found, the next step in the management is to perform a repeat test preferably after 3 months, to allow time for a complete cycle of spermatogenesis to take place. If the second test is also abnormal the next step is to perform FSH, LH, testosterone and prolactin levels and to assess the size of the testes, to determine whether the oligozoospermia is due to hypogonadotropic hypogonadism, hypergonadotropic hypogonadism or obstruction of the system of ducts. If the hormone levels are normal and the testicular volume is normal, the azoospermia is due to an obstructive cause. If FSH LH and testosterone levels are low, the failure is due to a hypothalamic or pituitary cause, or due to use of anabolic steroids. CT/MRI scan of the pituitary may be needed. If FSH and LH levels are high and the testicular volume is reduced, primary testicular failure is present.

Q. 5 (D)

Q. 6 (D)

Explanation for questions 5 and 6

Since the gonadotropin levels are low the oligozoospermia is due to hypogonadotropic hypogonadism. Since there is no intracranial lesion the next step in the management is to treat with clomiphene citrate 50 mg/day for 3 months. Since the treatment has resulted in some improvement, the next step in the management is hCG injections 1500 IU three times a week. If the response is not adequate, add HMG or FSH 75–150 IU intramuscularly 3 times per week, until an adequate response is obtained. There is no use in treating with tamoxifen as he has been treated with clomiphene. Artificial insemination with aspirated sperms is done only for obstructive causes. Artificial insemination with donor semen or *in vitro* fertilisation is indicated if treatment with gonadotropins fails.

Q. 7 (A)

Irrespective of the cause of oligozoospermia, the sperm concentration is adequate to consider artificial insemination, after preparation of the semen, as the first line treatment. If conception fails to occur after 3 cycles of treatment, the cause for the oligozoospermia should be sought and definitive treatment should be commenced.

Q. 8 (C)

Q. 9 (D)

Q. 9a (C)

Explanation for questions 8, 9 and 9a

This woman has long cycles and low serum progesterone levels indicating irregular ovulation. As she is not obese and the FSH and LH levels are low, she falls into the WHO group 1 ovulation disorders. Since the FSH and LH levels are in the low normal range, the first step in the management is to treat with clomiphene citrate and mid-cycle hCG injections. Clomiphene inhibits oestrogen receptors in the hypothalamus, inhibiting negative feedback of oestrogen on gonadotropin release. Since oestrogen can no longer effectively exert negative feedback on the hypothalamus, GnRH secretion becomes more rapidly pulsatile, which results in increased pituitary gonadotropin (FSH, LH) release. Increased FSH level causes growth of more ovarian follicles, with subsequent rupture of follicles resulting in ovulation. Ovulation occurs most often 6–7 days after a course of clomiphene. There is no need to perform follicular tracking prior to treatment, as anovulation is confirmed by low serum progesterone levels. However, follicular tracking should be performed during treatment cycles, to exclude ovarian hyperstimulation and to time the hCG injection, which should be given when the follicle is more than 1.8 cm. Ovulation is expected to occur 36 hours after the hCG injection.

If treatment with clomiphene citrate fails to restore ovulation and fertility, the next step in the management is to treat with FSH injections. The treatment is commenced on the third day of the cycle with daily injections of 75 IU. Transvaginal scanning is performed to determine the growth of the dominant follicle and to exclude ovarian hyperstimulation. If the dominant follicle does not reach 0.8 mm by the 7th day, the dose is gradually stepped up to a maximum of 150 IU. Treatment is continued till the follicle reaches 1.8 mm and hCG is given 36 hours before the estimated time of ovulation.

If there is no success with gonadotropins, the next step is pulsatile administration of GnRH using a pump. Monthly injections of GnRH are of no value.

Treatment with metformin or ovarian drilling is not indicated as there is no obesity or any other evidence of polycystic ovarian syndrome.

Q. 10 (D)

Q. 10a (B)

Explanation for questions 10 and 10a

This patient falls into WHO group 2 ovulation disorders. After advising weight reduction the first step is treatment with clomiphene citrate for 3 months. Since the patient is obese it is best to add metformin as well. If treatment with clomiphene and metformin fails, the next step is laparoscopic ovarian drilling as she has polycystic ovaries. Treating with FSH injections to induce follicular growth is an alternative.

Q. 11 (E)

Though the tubes are patent their function can be impaired due to peritubal adhesions. Since this woman has endometriosis as well, adhesiolysis and diathermy cauterisation of the endometriotic deposits should be done at the same time. *In vitro* fertilisation should be considered if the procedure does not result in a pregnancy. Intrauterine insemination and gamete intrafallopian transfer will not restore fertility if the tubal function is impaired.

Q. 12 (D)

Q. 13 (D)

Explanation for questions 12 and 13

Performing a seminal fluid analysis is the first step in investigating an infertile couple, because it is a non-invasive test and male factors are common causes of infertility. If the seminal fluid analysis is normal, the next step is to establish the occurrence of ovulation. A woman who has regular menstruation usually ovulates regularly. However, ovulation should be confirmed by performing day 21 progesterone level, which is a non-invasive test.

Q. 14 (B)

Since the seminal fluid analysis is normal and ovulation has been established, the next step is to confirm tubal patency. Hysterosalpingogram is a reliable test for tubal patency. It is less invasive and makes more efficient use of resources than laparoscopy. It is the best method to confirm tubal patency in this woman as she does not have co-morbidities, such as pelvic inflammatory disease, previous ectopic pregnancy, or endometriosis, which can be diagnosed and treated by laparoscopy. Tubal insufflation and hydrotubation are no longer regarded as accurate tests for tubal patency. Transvaginal scan is not a test for tubal patency. However, tubal patency tests are invasive procedures. Therefore, in most cases if there is no evidence of tubal pathology such as PID or endometriosis, tubal patency tests are performed only if the woman fails to conceive after preliminary treatment.

Q. 15 (C)

Since the seminal fluid analysis is normal and ovulation has been established the next step is to confirm tubal patency. Since this woman has frequent periods, dysmenorrhoea and dyspareunia, the cause of her infertility could be endometriosis. Laparoscopy is the appropriate test for tubal patency if other pelvic pathologies are suspected, as these can be diagnosed and treated at the same time.

Q. 16 (D)

A hysterosalpingogram should not be performed during menstruation as air embolism can occur. It should not be performed after day 11 because if ovulation and fertilisation occurs the embryo will be exposed to radiation. Therefore the most suitable period to perform a hysterosalpingogram is between days 7 and 11, when menstruation would have ceased and ovulation would not have occurred.

11

Early Pregnancy Failure

Miscarriage is a pregnancy loss under a gestational age of 24 weeks.

Types

- Threatened miscarriage
- Inevitable miscarriage
- Incomplete miscarriage
- Complete miscarriage
- Missed miscarriage/delayed miscarriage /anembryonic pregnancy/early foetal demise /blighted ovum

Definitions

- **Complete abortion:** All products of conception have been expelled, without the need for surgical or medical intervention.
- **Incomplete abortion:** Some, but not all, of the products of conception have been expelled. Retained products may be part of the foetus, placenta, or membranes.
- **Inevitable abortion:** The cervix has dilated with colicky lower abdominal pain, but the products of conception have not yet been expelled. However, the abortion cannot be prevented.
- **Missed abortion:** A pregnancy in which there is foetal demise (usually for a number of weeks), but there is no uterine activity to expel the products of conception.
- **Recurrent spontaneous abortions:** Three or more consecutive pregnancy losses.
- **Septic abortion:** A spontaneous abortion that is complicated by intrauterine infection.

- **Threatened abortion:** A pregnancy complicated with mild bleeding before 20 weeks gestation without an attempt to expel the foetus.

Causes

- Chromosomal abnormalities
  - Trisomies (Down's syndrome), Triploidies and tetraploidies (especially if the maternal age is more than 35 years).
  - Monosomy (Turner syndrome)
  - Hereditary translocations
- Endocrine disorders
  - Diabetes, hypothyroidism, luteal phase deficiency, polycystic ovarian syndrome
- Abnormalities of the uterus
  - Uterine septa (bicornuate uterus)
  - Endometrial adhesions
  - Cervical incompetence
- Infections
  - *Salmonella typhi*, malaria, cytomegalovirus, rubella, toxoplasmosis, *Chlamydia trachomatis*.
- Chemical agents
  - Tobacco, anaesthetic gases, arsenic, benzene, solvents, ethylene oxide, formaldehyde, pesticides, lead, mercury, cadmium.
- Immunological disorders
  - Antiphospholipid syndrome, thrombophilia (hereditary)

THREATENED MISCARRIAGE

Symptoms

- Period of amenorrhoea.
- Mild bleeding without passage of clots.
- Mild abdominal pain.

Examination Findings

- Cervical os will be closed.
- The size of the uterus will correspond to the period of amenorrhoea.

Investigations

- The serum beta hCG level will be appropriate for the period of amenorrhoea.
- The diagnosis is confirmed by ultrasound scanning. A live intrauterine pregnancy will be seen.

Treatment

- Reassurance is essential.
- The value of bedrest and administration of progesterone supplements is uncertain.
- Avoid sex until bleeding stops.
- Give anti-D to Rhesus negative women if bleeding occurs after 12 weeks.

INEVITABLE MISCARRIAGE

Symptoms

- Period of amenorrhoea.
- Profuse bleeding.
- Colicky lower abdominal pain.

Examination Findings

- Cervical os will be open and the products of conception will be felt at the os.
- The size of the uterus will correspond to the period of amenorrhoea.
- An inevitable miscarriage can proceed to become complete or incomplete depending on whether all products are expelled or not. The process cannot be reversed.
- The diagnosis is confirmed by the clinical picture.

- Investigations are of not much value to confirm the diagnosis.

Investigations

- The serum beta hCG level may be appropriate for the period of amenorrhoea.
- Ultrasound scanning may show a live intrauterine pregnancy.

Treatment

- The presence of products within the cervical canal can stimulate a vasovagal reflex, causing profuse bleeding and even shock.
- The first line treatment is to remove any products found within the cervical canal, using a sponge-holding forceps. This is carried out in the ward.
- If all the products cannot be removed and bleeding persists, insert vaginal misoprostol to complete the evacuation.
- Intravenous fluids and blood transfusion may be needed if the blood loss is excessive.
- Suction evacuation is done if the evacuation is not complete with medical management and the tissue thickness in the uterus is greater than 15 mm.

INCOMPLETE MISCARRIAGE

A period of amenorrhoea followed by intermittent, sometimes heavy bleeding and lower abdominal cramps.

Examination Findings

The cervical os is open and the size of the uterus is smaller than the period of amenorrhoea.

Investigations

The first step in the management is to perform a transvaginal ultrasound scan, to determine the amount of tissue left in the uterus.

Conservative Management

Conservative management is recommended in the absence of infection, if the anteroposterior diameter of the tissue within the endometrial cavity is less than 15 mm.

Ultrasound scans are performed once in two weeks till the uterus is empty.

Medical Management

- Medical management is recommended if the tissue thickness in the uterus is greater than 15 mm, or if bleeding persists for more than 15 days after conservative management.
- A single dose of 800 micrograms of misoprostol is inserted into the vagina.
- The patient should be reviewed if bleeding and expulsion of retained tissue does not occur within 24 hours.

Surgical Management

- Suction evacuation is done if the evacuation is not complete with medical management and the tissue thickness in the uterus is greater than 15 mm.
- The evacuated material is sent for histology to exclude GTD.

MISSED MISCARRIAGE/DELAYED MISCARRIAGE/BLIGHTED OVUM

Symptoms

A period of amenorrhoea which is followed by mild vaginal bleeding.

Examination Findings

The uterus will be smaller than the period of amenorrhoea and the cervical os will be closed.

Diagnosis

- The serum beta hCG level will be less than the expected value for the period of amenorrhoea and will continue to fall. If the levels fall by 50% in 48 hours, a missed miscarriage is more likely.
- Progesterone levels above 25 nmol/L are likely to indicate and above 60 nmol/L are strongly associated with an on-going pregnancy.
- The diagnosis is confirmed by the following findings on transvaginal ultrasound scanning.

- Mean gestational sac diameter (MGSD)> 25 mm with no foetal pole.
- Foetal pole >7 mm with no foetal heart pulsation.
- A repeat TVS performed at least 7 days from the original scan demonstrates a little or no change in the dimensions.

Do not use gestational age from the last menstrual period alone to determine whether a foetal heartbeat should be visible.

Treatment

Expectant Management

- This is the first line treatment

Medical Management

- It is indicated if expectant management fails in 7–14 days or if the patient refuses expectant management.
- A single dose of 800 micrograms of misoprostol is inserted into the vagina.

Suction Evacuation

- It is done if the evacuation is not complete with medical management and the tissue thickness in the uterus is greater than 15 mm.

Non-sensitised Rhesus negative women should receive prophylactic anti-D immunoglobulin in the following situations:

- Ectopic pregnancy.
- All miscarriages over 12 weeks gestation (including threatened).
- All miscarriages where the uterus is evacuated medically or surgically.
- Anti-D immunoglobulin should only be given for threatened miscarriage under 12 weeks gestation, when bleeding is heavy, recurrent or associated with pain.
- Anti-D is not required for cases of complete miscarriage under 12 weeks gestation, where there has been no medical or surgical intervention.

The Value of Ultrasound Scanning in the Diagnosis and Management of Early Pregnancy Failure and Ectopic Pregnancy

- A transvaginal scan is usually performed.
- The first ultrasound evidence of pregnancy is the gestational sac within the thickened decidua.
- 2–3 mm sac can be identified by 4 weeks and 2 days.
- The yolk sac is the first structure to be identified and should appear when the sac diameter is between 5 and 7 mm at 5 weeks.
- Presence of the foetal heart beat indicates a live embryo, but may not be seen until the embryo measures 5 mm at 6 weeks.
- If the foetal heart beat is not visible, identify the foetal pole and measure the crown-rump length.
- Measure the mean gestational sac diameter only if the foetal pole is not visible.
- If the crown-rump length is less than 7 mm and there is no visible heartbeat, repeat the scan after a minimum of 7 days.
- If the crown-rump length is more than 7 mm and there is no visible heartbeat, repeat the scan after a minimum of 7 days. There is a greater chance of a non-viable foetus.
- If a transabdominal scan is performed, repeat the scan after 14 days.
- If the mean gestational sac diameter is less than 25 mm with and there is no visible foetal pole, repeat the scan after 7 days.
- If the mean gestational sac diameter is more than 25 mm and there is no visible foetal pole, repeat the scan after 7 days. There is a greater chance of a non-viable foetus.
- If a transabdominal scan is performed, repeat the scan after 14 days.
- Do not use gestational age alone to determine whether a foetal heartbeat should be visible, as the date of the last menstrual period given by the woman may not be accurate, or the cycles may be long.

The Value of hCG Measurements in the Diagnosis and Management of Early Pregnancy Failure and Ectopic Pregnancy

- If serum or urine hCG is positive and there is no IUP on USS, always suspect an ectopic pregnancy, or a pregnancy in an unknown location. Do not diagnose a complete miscarriage unless there is a previous scan showing an IUP.
- Perform 2 serum beta hCG measurements 48 hours apart.
- If the rise is greater than 63%, a developing intrauterine pregnancy is most likely, although the possibility of an ectopic pregnancy cannot be completely excluded, till an IUP is seen on the USS. A repeat scan should be performed 7–14 days later.
- If the value decreases by more than 50%, a viable intrauterine pregnancy is unlikely.
- If there is a change in serum hCG concentration between a 50% decline and 63% rise, there is a high possibility of an ectopic pregnancy and further assessment at a specialised centre is required.

RECURRENT MISCARRIAGE

Recurrent miscarriage is defined as the loss of three or more consecutive pregnancies.

Causes

- Antiphospholipid syndrome:
  - It is the association between antiphospholipid antibodies (lupus anticoagulant, anticardiolipin antibodies and anti-B2 glycoprotein-I antibodies) and adverse pregnancy outcome or vascular thrombosis.
  - It is the most important treatable cause of recurrent miscarriage.
- Genetic factors
  - Parental chromosomal rearrangements—balanced translocations
  - Embryonic chromosomal abnormalities.
- Anatomical factors
  - Congenital uterine malformations.
  - Cervical incompetence.

- Endocrine factors
  - Poorly controlled diabetes mellitus.
  - Untreated thyroid disorders/presence of anti-thyroid antibodies
  - Polycystic ovary syndrome (may be due to insulin resistance, hyperinsulinaemia and increased androgen levels.)
- Immune factors
- Infective agents
  - For an infective agent to be implicated in the aetiology of repeated pregnancy loss, it must be capable of persisting in the genital tract and avoiding detection, by not causing symptoms to disturb the woman.
  - Toxoplasmosis, rubella, cytomegalo-virus, herpes and listeria infections do not fulfil these criteria and routine TORCH screening should be abandoned.
  - Bacterial vaginosis in the first trimester of pregnancy is regarded as a risk factor for second-trimester miscarriage and preterm delivery.
- Inherited thrombophilic defect.

INVESTIGATIONS

- Antiphospholipid antibodies
  - Prepregnancy testing should be done in women with a history of recurrent first-trimester miscarriages or one or more second-trimester miscarriages.
  - Antiphospholipid syndrome is diagnosed if the woman has two positive tests at least 12 weeks apart, for lupus anticoagulant or anticardiolipin anti-bodies of immunoglobulin G and/or immunoglobulin M class, present in a medium or high titre over 40 g/L, or above the 99th percentile.
- Karyotyping
  - Should be performed on products of conception of the third and subsequent consecutive miscarriages.
  - Should be performed in both partners of couples with recurrent miscarriages,

where an unbalanced structural chromo-somal abnormality is found, on testing the products of conception.
- Structural defects
  - Transvaginal ultrasound scan is performed.
  - Hysteroscopy and 3-dimensional ultra-sound scanning may be needed to confirm the diagnosis.
  - Serial transvaginal scanning is performed during the second trimester, to detect cervical shortening, if cervical incompetence is suspected.
- Thrombophilias
  - Screening for inherited thrombophilias, is necessary for women with a history of recurrent second-trimester miscarriages.

TREATMENT

Antiphospholipid Antibodies

- Treat with unfractionated or low molecular weight heparin and aspirin.
- Low molecular weight heparin is as safe as and has advantages over unfractionated heparin during pregnancy, since it causes less heparin-induced thrombocytopenia, can be administered once daily and is associated with a lower risk of heparin-induced osteoporosis.
- Heparin will improve the live birth rate in women with second trimester miscarriages due to inherited thrombophilia.

Genetic Abnormalities

- These patients should be referred for genetic screening.

Anatomical Defects

- Hysteroscopic resection may improve the outcome in cases of uterine septa.
- History indicated cervical circlage may be performed in women with 3 or more second trimester miscarriages or if the cervical

length is shorter than 25 mm on serial trans-vaginal scanning.

Endocrine and Immunological Effects

Supplementation with progesterone, human chorionic gonadotropins, suppression of high luteinising hormone levels among ovulatory women, metformin or intravenous immunoglobulin injections have not been confirmed to be beneficial in women with recurrent miscarriage

Unexplained miscarriages: Only need careful follow-up and reassurance.

REFERENCES

- Ectopic pregnancy and miscarriage: Diagnosis and initial management.
- The Investigation and Treatment of Couples with Recurrent First trimester and Second trimester Miscarriage. RCOG Green-top Guideline No. 17, April 2011.

QUESTIONS

1. A woman complains of sudden onset of colicky lower abdominal pain and profuse bleeding at a period of amenorrhoea of 10 weeks. She is pale and the blood pressure is 90/60 mmHg. The cervical os is open and products are felt at the os. Ultrasound scan reveals a live intrauterine pregnancy. Resuscitation is commenced.

   What is the next step in the management?

   A. Commence an infusion of oxytocin.
   B. Insert 600 mcg of misoprostol into the vagina.
   C. Perform an emergency cervical circlage.
   D. Perform an evacuation of retained products under general anaesthesia.
   E. Remove the products within the cervical canal with a sponge holding forceps.

2. A woman complains of sudden onset of colicky lower abdominal pain and profuse bleeding at a POA of 10 weeks. She is pale and the blood pressure is 90/60 mmHg. The cervical os is open and products are felt at the os. Resuscitation is commenced. Part of the products is removed from the cervical canal using a sponge holding forceps.

   What is the next step in the management?

   A. Commence an infusion of oxytocin.
   B. Give oral mifepristone.
   C. Insert 800 mcg of misoprostol into the vagina.
   D. Keep under observation for bleeding.
   E. Perform an evacuation of retained products under general anaesthesia.

3. A woman complains of mild lower abdominal pain and mild bleeding at a period of amenorrhoea of 8 weeks. The cervical os is closed and the size of the uterus corresponds to 8 weeks.

   What is the next step in the management?

   A. Administer progesterone supplements.
   B. Advise bedrest.
   C. Estimate serum beta hCG levels.
   D. Estimate serum progesterone levels.
   E. Perform an ultrasound scan.

4. A woman complains of mild lower abdominal pain and mild bleeding at a period of amenorrhoea of 8 weeks. The cervical os is closed and the size of the uterus corresponds to 8 weeks. Ultrasound scan reveals a live intrauterine pregnancy with a yolk sac.

   What is the most appropriate management?

A. Administer progesterone supplements.

B. Advise bedrest.

C. Administer mild analgesics.

D. Insert misoprostol if the serum β-hCG levels fall.

E. Reassurance and explanation only.

5. A woman complains of mild vaginal bleeding for one week at a period of amenorrhoea of 11 weeks. On vaginal examination the cervical os is closed and the uterine enlargement corresponds to 8 weeks.

What is the next step in the management?

A. Estimate serum beta hCG levels

B. Insert misoprostol into the vagina.

C. Perform a coagulation profile.

D. Perform an ultrasound scan.

E. Review after 10 days.

6. A woman complains of mild vaginal bleeding for one week at a period of amenorrhoea of 10 weeks. The cervical os is closed and the uterine enlargement corresponds to 8 weeks. Ultrasound scan reveals a 30 mm gestation sac with a foetal pole. The crown-rump length is 7 mm and there is no foetal heart beat.

What is the next step in the management?

A. Administer oral mifepristone.

B. Insert prostaglandin E2 into the vagina.

C. Insert misoprostol into the vagina.

D. Perform suction evacuation.

E. Repeat the ultrasound scan after one week.

7. A woman is complains of mild vaginal bleeding for one week at a period of amenorrhoea of 11 weeks. On vaginal examination the cervical os is closed and the uterine enlargement corresponds to 8 weeks. Two ultrasound scans performed one week apart confirm a missed abortion.

What is the most appropriate first step in the management?

A. Administer oral mifepristone.

B. Administer vaginal prostaglandin E2 tablets.

C. Carry out expectant management for one week.

D. Commence an infusion of oxytocin.

E. Insert misoprostol into the vagina.

8. A woman complains of mild vaginal bleeding for one week at a period of amenorrhoea of 11 weeks. The cervical os is closed and the uterine enlargement corresponds to 8 weeks. Ultrasound scan confirms a missed abortion. She refuses expectant management.

What is the most appropriate management?

A. Administer vaginal prostaglandin E2 tablets.

B. Commence an infusion of oxytocin.

C. Insert 800 mcg of misoprostol into the vagina.

D. Perform a dilatation and evacuation.

E. Perform a suction evacuation.

9. A woman is admitted with a history of profuse vaginal bleeding with clots, followed by continuous mild vaginal bleeding for one week at a period of amenorrhoea of 10 weeks. The cervical os is open and the uterine enlargement corresponds to 8 weeks. Ultrasound scan reveals an endometrial thickness of 25 mm but no gestation sac.

What is the most appropriate management?

A. Administer oral mifepristone

B. Insert misoprostol into the vagina.

C. Perform dilatation and curettage.

D. Perform suction evacuation.

E. Repeat the ultrasound scan in one week.

10. A routine transvaginal scan is performed on a woman who attends the antenatal clinic at a POA of 6 weeks. An intrauterine gestational sac with a foetal pole is identified. The crown-rump length is 5 mm. The foetal heartbeat is not seen. She has no complaints.

What is the next step in the management?

A. Estimate serum beta hCG.

B. Obtain an accurate menstrual history from the patient.

C. Perform 2 serum beta hCG measurements 48 hours apart.

D. Perform a repeat transvaginal scan in 14 days.

E. Perform a repeat transvaginal scan in 7 days.

10a. A routine transvaginal scan is performed on a woman who attends the antenatal clinic at a POA of 10 weeks. An intrauterine gestational sac with a foetal pole is identified. The crown-rump length is 8 mm. The foetal heart beat is not seen. She has no complaints.

What is the next step in the management?

A. Commence an infusion of oxytocin.

B. Insert vaginal misoprostol.

C. Perform 2 serum hCG measurements 48 hours apart.

D. Perform a repeat transvaginal scan in 14 days.

E. Perform a repeat transvaginal scan in 7 days.

11. A woman complains of abdominal pain and scanty vaginal bleeding at a POA of 6 weeks. She has 28-day regular cycles. The urine pregnancy test is positive. A transvaginal ultrasound scan is performed. An intrauterine gestational sac is not identified.

What is the next step in the management?

A. Estimate serum beta hCG levels.

B. Obtain an accurate menstrual history from the patient.

C. Perform two serum beta hCG measurements 48 hours apart.

D. Perform a laparoscopy.

E. Perform a repeat transvaginal scan in 7 days.

12. A woman who has had 3 previous first trimester miscarriages attends the antenatal clinic at a period of amenorrhoea of 5 weeks. She is positive for lupus anticoagulant and anti-phospholipid antibodies.

What is the best management?

A. Treat with aspirin after 12th week.

B. Treat with low molecular weight heparin during the first trimester and warfarin during the second and third trimesters.

C. Treat with low molecular weight heparin if the coagulation profile is abnormal.

D. Treat with low molecular weight heparin throughout the pregnancy.

E. Treat with unfractionated heparin throughout the pregnancy.

13. A woman who has had 2 previous second trimester miscarriages between the 18th and the 22nd weeks attends the antenatal clinic at a period of amenorrhoea of 12 weeks.

What is the best management option?

A. Insert a cervical circlage at 12 weeks.

B. Insert a cervical circlage at 16 weeks.

C. Insert a cervical circlage if the cervical length is less than 25 mm.

D. Treat with oral nifedepine till 28 weeks.

E. Treat with oral progestogen till 24 weeks.

ANSWERS AND EXPLANATIONS

Q. 1 (E)

Q. 2 (C)

Explanation for questions 1 and 2

A diagnosis of an inevitable abortion can be made, because she is having colicky abdominal pain with profuse bleeding. Also the cervical os is open, products can be felt at the os and a live pregnancy is seen on the ultrasound scan.

The presence of products within the cervical canal can stimulate a vasovagal reflex, causing profuse bleeding and even shock. Therefore, the first step in the management is removal of the products found in the cervical canal, using a sponge holding forceps. This is done in the ward and it will reduce the bleeding and shock. However, in most cases this initial evacuation will be incomplete and misoprostol should be inserted to complete the evacuation. Evacuation of retained products under general anaesthesia is necessary only if the evacuation is not completed after insertion of misoprostol. Once an abortion is inevitable it cannot be prevented by performing a cervical circlage. Oxytocin is less effective than misoprostol in first and second trimester miscarriages.

Q. 3 (E)

Q. 4 (E)

Explanation for questions 3 and 4

The most probable diagnosis is threatened abortion, because she has a period of amenorrhoea followed by mild pain and mild bleeding. The cervical os is closed and the size of the uterus corresponds to the period of amenorrhoea.

The next step is to perform an ultrasound scan to confirm the diagnosis, by the presence of a live pregnancy with a yolk sac. Serum beta hCG levels will be appropriate for the POA and will double in 48 hours. Progesterone levels above 25 nmol/L are likely to indicate and above 60 nmol/L are strongly associated with a continuing live pregnancy. However, visualisation of a live foetus and the yolk sac by ultrasound scanning is the most reliable method to confirm the diagnosis.

Once the diagnosis is confirmed, the most appropriate option is to reassure and explain to the patient, that if the pregnancy continues, the foetus is unlikely to be affected and that there is no definite treatment. The pregnancy is most likely to continue unharmed, as the yolk sac is intact and there is no choriodecidual bleeding. Bedrest and progesterone supplements are of a little value. However, it is better to avoid strenuous exercise and sexual intercourse.

Q. 5 (D)

Q. 6 (E)

Q. 7 (C)

Q. 8 (C)

Explanation for questions 5, 6, 7 and 8

This patient most probably has a missed abortion as she has mild vaginal bleeding and the uterus is smaller than the period of amenorrhoea with a closed os. The next step in the management is to perform an ultrasound scan. The diagnosis is suspected by the presence of a 30 mm gestation sac, with a foetal pole of 7 mm, without a foetal heart beat.

The next step is to repeat the scan in one week, to confirm the diagnosis by the persistent absence of the foetal heart beat.

The best management option is to observe for 7–14 days, for spontaneous expulsion to occur. If the patient is not willing for expectant management or if expectant management fails, the next step is to insert vaginal misoprostol to stimulate expulsion. Oxytocin, mifepristone and prostaglandine E2 are not effective in the first trimester.

Q. 9 (B)

A diagnosis of an incomplete miscarriage is made, because there is continuous bleeding, following an abortion. The cervical os is open and the size of the uterus is less than the period of amenorrhoea. Medical evacuation with misoprostol is the most appropriate treatment, because there is continuous bleeding and the endometrial thickness is greater than 15 mm. The evacuated material is sent for histology, to exclude gestational trophoblastic tumour.

Surgical evacuation is indicated if:

- there is infection,
- medical management fails,
- there is an increased risk of bleeding,
- gestational trophoblastic disease is suspected.

Q. 10 (E); Q. 10a (E)

Explanation for questions 10 and 10a

The foetal heart beat should be visible by 6 weeks if the gestational age is correct. However, since the CRL is less than 7 mm, the next step in the management is to repeat the transvaginal scan in 7 days. Gestational age alone should not be used to determine whether the foetal heartbeat should be visible, as the date of the last menstrual period given by the woman may not be accurate or the cycles may be long.

When the POA is more than 6 weeks, or the crown-rump length is more than 7 mm, the foetal heartbeat should be visible. However, if the heartbeat is not seen, the next step is to repeat the TVUS after 7 days. There is a greater chance of a non-viable foetus in this case. The diagnosis of a nonviable pregnancy is confirmed and treatment is commenced only after the second scan.

Q. 11 (C)

If urine hCG is positive and there is no IUP on the USS, always suspect an ectopic pregnancy, or a pregnancy in an unknown location. Do not diagnose a complete or an incomplete miscarriage unless there is a previous scan showing an IUP. The next step in the management is to perform 2 serum beta hCG measurements 48 hours apart. If the rise is greater than 63%, a developing intrauterine pregnancy is most likely, although the possibility of an ectopic pregnancy cannot be completely excluded, till an IUP is seen on the USS. A repeat scan should be performed 7–14 days later. If the value decreases by more than 50%, a viable intrauterine pregnancy is unlikely. If there is a change in serum hCG concentration between a 50% decline and 63% rise, there is a high possibility of an ectopic pregnancy. A laparoscopy should be performed in this situation to exclude an ectopic pregnancy.

Q. 12 (D)

Women with recurrent first trimester miscarriages due to antiphospholipid antibodies should be treated with unfractionated or low molecular weight heparin. Low molecular weight heparin is as safe as and has advantages over unfractionated heparin during pregnancy, since it causes less heparin-induced thrombocytopenia, can be administered once daily and is associated with a lower risk of heparin-induced osteoporosis. Therefore, it is the best option for this patient. Aspirin can also be added from 14 weeks but aspirin alone is not effective.

Q. 13 (C)

A history indicated cervical circlage is performed if a woman gives a history of 3 or more recurrent second trimester miscarriages. This woman has had only 2 second trimester miscarriages. Therefore, serial transvaginal ultrasound scans should be done every 2 weeks during the second trimester and a circlage should be inserted only if the cervical length is less than 25 mm. Oral nifedipine and oral progestogen are not given to prevent second trimester miscarriages.

12

Ectopic Pregnancy

Symptoms

- A period of amenorrhoea between 4 and 12 weeks
  - The usual time of presentation is between 6 and 10 weeks.
  - An ectopic in the isthmus of the tube can rupture as early as 4 weeks, while a cornual ectopic can go up to 12 weeks or longer.
- Abdominal pain
  - Sudden onset of pain is more common with a ruptured ectopic, while an aching pain may be present in a chronic ectopic.
  - Pain is always the prominent symptom.
- Fainting attacks.
- Vaginal bleeding.
- Other symptoms
  - Shoulder tip pain, urinary symptoms.

Signs

- General condition:
  - will be poor with pallor, tachycardia and low blood pressure if rupture has occurred.
  - will be satisfactory in unruptured and chronic cases.
- Abdomen:
  - Tenderness may be present.
  - Guarding, rigidity and distension will be present if rupture has occurred.
- Vaginal examination:
  - Will be helpful but is not essential for the diagnosis.
  - Should be done in a hospital as the procedure can cause rupture.
  - There will be acute tenderness in the adnexa.
  - Cervical motion tenderness may be present.
  - An adnexal mass may be felt.

Diagnosis

- Ectopic pregnancy should be suspected in a woman of childbearing age, who complains of abdominal pain, even in the absence of a POA.
- Usually an ectopic pregnancy is suspected by the presence of a POA, abdominal pain and bleeding. The above mentioned physical signs will be helpful in the diagnosis.
- The next step in the diagnosis is to perform a transvaginal ultrasound scan.
- If an ectopic pregnancy or an IUP is not identified by the scan, perform serum beta hCG levels and repeat the test and the transvaginal scan in 48 hours.

- If the level plateaus shows a rise of less than 63% and there is no IUP, an ectopic pregnancy/pregnancy in an unknown location is suspected.
- Laparoscopy should be performed in these cases to confirm the diagnosis and for management.
- If the serum beta hCG level rises by more than 63% or doubles, a developing IUP should be confirmed by performing a TVUS in 3–7 days.
- If the level falls by more than 50%, a diagnosis of a nonviable pregnancy is made.

Transvaginal Ultrasound Scan

Following ultrasound features can be used to diagnose an ectopic pregnancy.

- Absence of an intrauterine pregnancy.
- Positive identification of an inhomogenous mass, empty adnexal gestation sac or an adnexal sac containing a yolk sac or a foetal pole.
- Presence of free fluid in the peritoneal cavity is suggestive of an ectopic pregnancy in the absence of an IUP, but not diagnostic, as a small amount may be physiological.

Treatment

Medical treatment with methotrexate is the first line treatment for an unruptured ectopic pregnancy:

- where the patient consents for medical treatment,
- with an adnexal mass smaller than 35 mm with no visible heartbeat,
- with a serum β-hCG level less than 1500 IU/L,
- where there is no significant pain,
- where the patient is able to come for regular follow-up.

All the above criteria should be satisfied.

Single Dose Methotrexate Regimen

Day 1: Administer a single dose of intramuscular methotrexate, 50 mg per m^2

Days 4 and 7: Measure β-hCG level.

Repeat the dose if the decrease in β-hCG level is less than 15% between days 4 and 7.

After initial treatment response, measure β-hCG level weekly until it reaches zero.

Surgical treatment is the first-line treatment for:

- women who are not willing for medical treatment,
- women who are unable to return for follow-up,
- an ectopic pregnancy with significant pain,
- an ectopic pregnancy with an adnexal mass of 35 mm or larger,
- an ectopic pregnancy with a foetal heart beat visible on the ultrasound scan,
- an ectopic pregnancy with a serum hCG level of 5000 IU/L or more.
- a ruptured ectopic pregnancy.

Surgical Treatment

- Immediate surgery is indicated for a ruptured ectopic pregnancy.
- If the patient is haemodynamically unstable quick resuscitation is carried out.
- Laparoscopy is the gold standard for diagnosis and treatment especially if a ruptured ectopic pregnancy is suspected.
- However, laparoscopy should be avoided and a laparotomy should be performed in a haemodynamically unstable/collapsed patient.
- Salpingectomy is the most appropriate surgical procedure.
- Salpingotomy is done in women with contralateral tube damage.
- Serum hCG is measured 1 week after surgery and then weekly until a negative result is obtained.

QUESTIONS

1. A 20-year-old woman complains of sudden onset of right-sided lower abdominal pain and bleeding per vagina. Her last normal menstrual period was 35 days ago. Her blood pressure is 90/70 mmHg and the pulse rate is 100 bpm. There is tenderness and guarding in the right iliac fossa. She denies any sexual intercourse.

   What is the most appropriate next step in the management?
   A. Estimate serum beta hCG levels.
   B. Obtain a surgical opinion to exclude acute appendicitis.
   C. Perform a laparoscopic examination.
   D. Perform a transvaginal ultrasound scan.
   E. Perform a urine hCG test.

2. A thirdpara is admitted with a history of sudden onset of right-sided lower abdominal pain and bleeding per vagina after a period of amenorrhoea of 5 weeks. Her blood pressure is 90/70 mmHg and the pulse rate is 110 bpm. Transvaginal ultrasound scan reveals the presence of a large amount of free fluid in the pelvis and the absence of an intrauterine pregnancy.

   What is the most appropriate management?
   A. Perform laparoscopic salpingectomy.
   B. Perform laparoscopic salpingo-oophorectomy.
   C. Perform laparoscopic salpingotomy.
   D. Perform a salpingectomy through a laparotomy.
   E. Treat with intramuscular methotrexate.

2a. A thirdpara complains of sudden onset of right-sided lower abdominal pain and bleeding per vagina after a period of amenorrhoea of 6 weeks. Her blood pressure is 80/50 mmHg and the pulse rate is 130 bpm. Transvaginal ultrasound scan reveals a large amount of free fluid in the pelvis and the absence of an intrauterine pregnancy. Resuscitation is commenced

   What is the most appropriate management?
   A. Perform a laparoscopic salpingectomy.
   B. Perform a laparoscopic salpingo-oophorectomy.
   C. Perform a salpingectomy through a laparotomy.
   D. Perform a salpingotomy through a laparotomy.
   E. Treat with intramuscular methotrexate.

3. A woman complains of right-sided lower abdominal pain and mild bleeding per vagina for one day after a period of amenorrhoea of 6 weeks. Her general condition is satisfactory. There is tenderness in the right iliac fossa. The urine hCG test is positive.

   What is the most appropriate next step in the management?
   A. Estimate serum beta hCG levels.
   B. Perform a transvaginal ultrasound scan.
   C. Perform a full blood count.
   D. Perform a transabdominal ultrasound scan.
   E. Review after one week

4. A woman complains of right-sided lower abdominal pain and mild bleeding per vagina for one day after a period of amenorrhoea of 6 weeks. Her general condition is satisfactory. There is tenderness in the right iliac fossa. The urine hCG test is positive. Transvaginal ultrasound scan does not reveal an adnexal mass or an intrauterine pregnancy.

   What is the next step in the management?

A. Commence treatment with metho-trexate.
B. Perform a laparoscopic examination.
C. Perform a single serum beta hCG test.
D. Perform two serum beta hCG tests 48 hours apart.
E. Repeat the ultrasound scan after 7 days.

5. A woman complains of right-sided lower abdominal pain and mild bleeding per vagina after a POA of 6 weeks. Her general condition is satisfactory. The urine hCG test is positive. Transvaginal ultrasound scan reveals an adnexal mass 30 mm in diameter without evidence of cardiac activity, but no intrauterine pregnancy.
   What is the most appropriate management?
   A. Perform laparoscopic salpingectomy.
   B. Perform laparoscopic salpingo-oophorectomy.
   C. Perform laparoscopic salpingotomy.
   D. Perform salpingectomy through a laparotomy.
   E. Treat with intramuscular methotrexate.

6. A woman complains of right-sided lower abdominal pain and mild bleeding per vagina after a period of amenorrhoea of 6 weeks. Her general condition is satisfactory. The urine hCG test is positive. An intrauterine pregnancy or an adnexal mass is not seen on the transvaginal ultrasound scan. Two serum beta hCG levels done 48 hours apart show an increase of 55%.
   What is the most appropriate management?
   A. Keep under observation for a further period of 7 days.
   B. Perform a diagnostic laparotomy.
   C. Perform a laparoscopy.
   D. Perform serial transvaginal ultrasound scans.
   E. Treat with a single dose of intramuscular methotrexate.

7. A woman attends the antenatal clinic at a POA of 5 weeks. She has no complaints. Her periods are regular and she is sure of dates. Urine hCG is positive. Transvaginal scan does not reveal an intrauterine or ectopic pregnancy. Serum beta hCG doubles from 900 to 1800 IU/L after 48 hours.
   What is the next step in the management?
   A. Give a single dose of methotrexate.
   B. Perform a laparoscopy.
   C. Perform a serum beta hCG test after 1 week.
   D. Reassure and review in the clinic after one month.
   E. Repeat the transvaginal scan in 3 days.

ANSWERS AND EXPLANATIONS

Q. 1 (D)

A provisional diagnosis of ruptured ectopic pregnancy can be made because she has a very short period of amenorrhoea, followed by abdominal pain and bleeding, together with tachycardia, low blood pressure, abdominal tenderness and guarding. An ectopic pregnancy should be suspected in a woman of child bearing age who presents with the above symptoms even in the absence of a POA. As her haemodynamic condition is fairly stable, the next step in the management is to perform a transvaginal ultrasound scan, to confirm the diagnosis by the absence of an intrauterine pregnancy and presence of free fluid in the peritoneal cavity. Estimation of serum beta hCG levels is of a little value, when a ruptured ectopic pregnancy is suspected, because the diagnosis can be confirmed only after repeating the test in 48 hours.

Q. 2 (A)

A diagnosis of a ruptured ectopic pregnancy can be suspected by the clinical picture. The diagnosis is confirmed by demonstrating free fluid and absence of an IUP on the transvaginal scan. The most appropriate management of a ruptured ectopic pregnancy is laparoscopic salpingectomy. Salpingotomy is done only in women with contralateral tubal damage. There is no place for medical management with methotrexate, in the treatment of a ruptured ectopic pregnancy.

Q. 2a (C)

As this patient is haemodynamically unstable, a quick diagnosis of a ruptured ectopic pregnancy should be made clinically and confirmed by performing a transvaginal ultrasound scan. Resuscitation and surgery should be undertaken simultaneously and immediately. A surgical procedure which prevents further blood loss most quickly should be used. In most centres laparotomy is carried out in a patient with a ruptured ectopic pregnancy who is haemodynamically unstable.

Q. 3 (B) and Q. 4 (D)

Explanation for questions 3 and 4
Since this woman has abdominal pain and bleeding after a POA of 6 weeks, with positive urine hCG test, a miscarriage or an ectopic pregnancy should be suspected. The next step in the management is to perform a transvaginal scan. If an ectopic or an IUP is not seen, a pregnancy in an unknown location should be suspected. The next step is to perform two serum beta hCG tests 48 hours apart. If the level plateaus, or if there is a rise of less than 63%, an ectopic pregnancy should be suspected and a laparoscopy should be done. It is not advisable to wait for 7 days to perform a repeat scan, as rupture could occur if an ectopic pregnancy is present.

Q. 5 (E)

Medical treatment is an option, when an ectopic pregnancy has been diagnosed with ultrasonography, as in this case, without the need for laparoscopy. Medical treatment with methotrexate is the best option for this patient, as she has an adnexal mass less than 35 mm in diameter, without cardiac activity and her general condition is stable. The patient should agree to come for regular and frequent follow-up visits.

Q. 6 (C)

In this case a diagnosis of a pregnancy in an unknown location is made, because there is a 55% increase in the serum β-hCG in 48 hours, but no IUP or an ectopic pregnancy is seen on the ultrasound scan. Since the diagnosis or the site of the pregnancy is not confirmed, the best management option is to perform a laparoscopy, for the diagnosis and treatment. It is safer than observation for 7 days, as the patient may not come for follow-up and sudden rupture can occur, if an ectopic pregnancy is present. Medical treatment can be considered only if an unruptured ectopic pregnancy has been diagnosed by ultrasound scanning.

Q. 7 (E)

This woman has a positive urine hCG test, but the TVUS does not reveal an IUP or an ectopic pregnancy. Therefore, her POA could be less than 5 weeks, or she could be having a pregnancy in an unknown location. Serum beta hCG levels doubled up to 1800 IU/L in 48 hours. Accordingly she is likely to have a developing early intrauterine pregnancy with wrong dates, but the possibility of an ectopic pregnancy cannot be excluded, as an IUP was not seen. The next step in the management is to perform a repeat TVUS. However the scan should be performed in 3 days, as the serum beta hCG is more than 1500 IU/L and there is the risk of rupture if a tubal pregnancy is present. (This is the case history of a patient who had a tubal abortion 3 days after the beta hCG test.)

REFERENCE

• Ectopic pregnancy and miscarriage: Diagnosis and initial management, NICE guidelines [CG154], December 2012.

13

Gestational Trophoblastic Disease

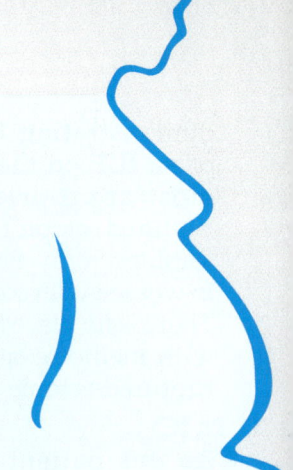

Definition

Gestational trophoblastic disease (GTD) form a spectrum of diseases extending from the benign conditions of complete and partial molar pregnancies to the malignant conditions of invasive mole, choriocarcinoma, placental site trophoblastic tumour (PSTT) and epithelioid trophoblastic tumour (ETT).

The spectrum of trophoblastic disease (FIGO Classification)

Benign	Hydatidiform mole
	Complete mole
	Partial mole
Clinically malignant	Invasive mole
Neoplastic	Choriocarcinoma
	PSTT
	ETT

Gestational trophoblastic neoplasia (GTN) includes:

- persistent postmolar gestational trophoblastic disease,
- invasive hydatidiform mole,
- choriocarcinoma,
- placental site trophoblastic tumour (PSTT),
- epithelioid trophoblastic tumour (ETT).

Risk factors for the occurrence of gestational trophoblastic neoplasia

- Extremes of reproductive age—under 20 years or over 40 years.
- Previous history of a molar pregnancy.
- Blood group A women married to blood group O men.
- Diet low in vitamin A.

HYDATIDIFORM MOLE

- There is abnormal proliferation and oedema of chorionic villi and stroma.
- Rapidly proliferating trophoblast secretes large amounts of hCG.
- It is divided into partial and complete molar pregnancies, depending on the presence or absence of foetal embryonic tissue, histopathological examination findings and on genetic features.
- Large theca-lutein cysts of the ovaries occur due to hyperstimulation with hCG.

Complete Moles

- Consist of swollen chorionic villi devoid of foetal blood vessels with atypical growth and proliferation of villous trophoblast
- Have no evidence of foetal tissue
- Are diploid and paternal in origin. Karyotype is 46XX (90%) or 46XY(10%)
- Usually (75–80%) arise due to duplication of a single sperm following fertilisation of an 'empty' ovum
- About 20–25% arises after dispermic fertilisation of an 'empty' ovum

- The maternal chromosomes may be either inactivated or absent, remaining only inside the mitochondria.

Partial Moles

- Vesicular changes occur only in a part of the villous population (focal rather than diffuse).
- There is scalloping of chorionic villi.
- They are usually (90%) triploid in origin, with two sets of paternal haploid genes and one set of maternal haploid genes. The karyotype is 69XXX or 69XXY.
- They occur following dispermic fertilisation of an ovum.
- 10% of partial moles represent tetraploid or mosaic conceptions.
- There may be a foetus or embryonic tissue or amnion or foetal red blood cells.

INVASIVE HYDATIDIFORM MOLE

- Includes 5 to 10% of moles (mainly complete rarely partial).
- The villi invade the myometrium but only about 15% spread outside the uterus
- It is not a malignant lesion. It is the molar version of placenta increta.

CHORIOCARCINOMA

- Is a malignant neoplasm of trophoblast.
- Spread occurs at an early stage to brain, lungs, liver, kidney and gastrointestinal tract.

Clinical Presentation of a Molar Pregnancy

- A period of amenorrhoea followed by vaginal bleeding is the commonest presenting symptom.
- The diagnosis can be clinically confirmed if there is passage of vesicles.
- Hyperemesis gravidarum.
- Excessive uterine enlargement (may not be found in partial moles)

- Rare presentations (not found in partial moles)
  - Hyperthyroidism
  - Early onset pre-eclampsia
  - Abdominal distension due to theca-lutein cysts

DIAGNOSIS

- Clinical symptoms and signs.
- Passage of vesicles.
- Increased hCG level greater than two multiples of the median. However, there is no consensus on a cut-off level. Pre-evacuation hCG is used as a baseline for follow-up.
- Pre-evacuation diagnosis is confirmed by USS.
  - Accuracy of ultrasound diagnosis increases with the gestational age.
  - Characteristic snowstorm appearance is found in a complete mole.
  - Bilateral theca-lutein cysts may be present.
- Diagnosis is more difficult in partial moles. Pre-evacuation clinical and ultrasound diagnosis is usually a missed or incomplete abortion.
- A chest X-ray should be done in complete moles to exclude lung metastases.

Histological Diagnosis

- Definitive diagnosis of hydatidiform mole is by histology.
- Histopathological examination is the only method to arrive at a definite diagnosis of some cases of partial moles. Therefore, histological examination of material obtained from medical or surgical evacuation of all failed pregnancies, is recommended to exclude trophoblastic neoplasia.
- Histological examination is essential in all repeat evacuations and in postpartum evacuations.
- Histological examination is not necessary following therapeutic termination of

pregnancy, if foetal parts have been identified on prior ultrasound scanning.

- Karyotyping and immunohistochemistry staining for P57 could be used to differentiate partial from complete moles.

TREATMENT

- Profuse bleeding can occur during evacuation. 3 pints of blood should be crossmatched.
- Suction evacuation is the method of choice for evacuation of complete molar pregnancies, as it minimises the risk of trophoblastic embolization.
- Cervical preparation with misoprostol or prostaglandin should be avoided to prevent trophoblastic embolization.
- Oxytocin should not be commenced till the evacuation is complete.
- If significant bleeding occurs during evacuation, it should be expedited and need for oxytocin should be weighed up against the risk of trophoblastic embolization.
- Suction evacuation is the method of choice for evacuation of partial molar pregnancies, except when the size of the foetal parts precludes its use. Medical evacuation is recommended for these patients. However, there is an increased risk of persistent trophoblastic disease.
- Routine second uterine evacuation is not recommended. If symptoms persist, serum hCG levels and ultrasound scanning should be done.
- Because of poor vascularisation of the chorionic villi and absence of the anti-D antigen in complete moles, anti-D prophylaxis is not required. It is, however, required for partial moles. However, anti-D is given following evacuation of all molar pregnancies, as most of the partial moles are diagnosed only later, by histological examination.
- Theca-lutein cysts regress and disappear following evacuation.
- Hysterectomy is the treatment of choice for women over the age of 40 years, especially if there are other risk factors such as large theca-lutein cysts, significant uterine enlargement, or pre-treatment hCG level more than 10^5.

Follow-up

- After histological confirmation of a molar pregnancy, hCG levels are estimated once a week, until the levels return to normal.
- If the hCG levels return to normal within 56 days after evacuation, hCG levels will be checked monthly for 6 months from the day of evacuation.
- If the hCG levels return to normal more than 56 days after evacuation, hCG levels will be checked monthly for 6 months after the values become normal.
- Women should be advised not to conceive till their follow-up is complete. Women who need chemotherapy should not conceive for 1 year after the treatment is complete.
- A reliable contraceptive method should be used for at least 6 months after the hCG level becomes normal.
- If the hCG level is normal any method can be used. If hCG is elevated a barrier method should be used.
- There is a 1–2% risk of recurrence of the disease in future pregnancies. Therefore, an early ultrasound scan should be performed. hCG levels should be measured 6–8 weeks after the end of any future pregnancy (whatever the outcome) to exclude disease recurrence.

GESTATIONAL TROPHOBLASTIC NEOPLASIA

- The abnormal trophoblast cells continue to be active and undergo proliferation in about 15% of cases of complete molar pregnancies and 0.5% of cases of partial molar pregnancies. This can metastasize.
- There is no reliable diagnostic tool to determine how a molar pregnancy will behave after evacuation and whether further treatment will be required.
- However, serial measurement of hCG levels give a very accurate assessment of the level of disease activity.

- Any woman who develops persistent or irregular vaginal bleeding following a pregnancy event should be suspected of having GTN. A urine pregnancy test should be performed in women who develop abnormal vaginal bleeding after a pregnancy event. Symptoms of metastasis, such as dyspnoea or neurological signs, occur very rarely.
- The change in diagnosis from a premalignant molar pregnancy, to a malignant form of gestational trophoblastic neoplasia which requires chemotherapy, is usually made clinically.
- Further biopsies are rarely performed.

Diagnosis Based on Clinical Assessment and Pattern of Change in hCG Levels

- Irregular vaginal bleeding.
- Rising hCG levels.
- hCG plateau in 3 consecutive samples.
- A hCG level of more than 20000 IU/L 4 weeks after evacuation.
- Raised hCG level 6 months after evacuation.
- Histological evidence of choriocarcinoma.
- Evidence of distant organ metastasis

Treatment

- Patients with scores of 6 or less are at low risk. They are treated with a single drug.
- Methotrexate 50 mg intramuscularly (or 1 mg/kg) is given every other day for 4 days, with leucovorin 15 mg (or 0.1 mg/kg) 24–30 hours after each dose of methotrexate. The course is repeated after 6 rest days till the serum hCG becomes negative.
- Women with scores of 7 or more are at high risk. They need treatment with multiple chemotherapeutic drugs.
- The drugs which are used include combinations of intravenous methotrexate, dactinomycin, etoposide, cyclophosphamide and vincristine, with folinic acid rescue.
- A hysterectomy should be done if the focus is in the uterus and the woman does not desire further pregnancies.
- Treatment should be continued for 6 weeks after the hCG level becomes normal. The cure rate for women with a score ≤6 is almost 100%; the rate for women with a score ≥7 is 95%.
- hCG is done twice weekly during treatment.
- Once hCG is normal treatment is continued for another 6 weeks.

Table 13.1: Proposed FIGO 2000 scoring system for gestational trophoblastic disease

Prognostic factors	Score[a]			
	0	1	2	4
Age (yr)	≤39	>39		
Antecedent pregnancy	Hydatidiform mole	Abortion	Term	
Interval (mo)[b]	<4	4–6	7–12	>12
hCG (IU/L)	<1,000	1,000–10,000	10,000–100,000	>100,000
Largest tumour	<3 cm	3–4 cm	≥5 cm	
Site(s) of metastases	Lung	Spleen, kidney	GI tract, liver	Brain
Number of metastases		1–3	4–8	>8
Prior chemotherapy			Single drug	Two or more drugs

[a] The total score for a patient is obtained by adding the individual scores of each prognostic factor; 4 or less = low risk, 5–7 = intermediate risk, > 7 = high risk.

[b] Time between end of antecedent pregnancy and start of chemotherapy.
  Adapted with permission from Kohorn EI, Goldstein DP, Hancock BW, et al.; Int J Gynecol Cancer 10:84–88, 2000.

- After normalization, hCG levels are done weekly for 6 weeks and two weekly for 12 weeks. Finally urine hCG is done after 6 months.

- Avoid pregnancy for 12 months after completion of chemotherapy to avoid misinterpretation of hCG and to avoid harmful effects of chemotherapy on the pregnancy.

QUESTIONS

1. A woman complains of excessive vomiting and mild vaginal bleeding for 5 days at a period of amenorrhoea of 10 weeks. The fundal height corresponds to 14 weeks.

   Which of the following is the most appropriate test to diagnose a molar pregnancy in this patient?

   A. Demonstrate the absence of foetal heart sounds using a hand Doppler.
   B. Perform a urine hCG test.
   C. Perform a single serum beta hCG level.
   D. Perform an ultrasound scan.
   E. Perform serial estimations of beta hCG levels.

2. A 30-year-old woman complains of excessive vomiting and mild vaginal bleeding for two weeks, at a POA of 12 weeks. The fundal height corresponds to 16 weeks. The cervical os is closed. Ultrasound scan demonstrates a snowstorm appearance in the uterus with no foetal parts.

   What is the best management option?

   A. Commence an oxytocin infusion after cervical priming with misoprostol.
   B. Perform suction evacuation and repeat the procedure after two weeks.
   C. Perform suction evacuation.
   D. Perform suction evacuation after commencing an oxytocin infusion.
   E. Perform suction evacuation after giving oral mifepristone.

3. A 30-year-old woman complains of vaginal bleeding for two weeks at a POA of 10 weeks. A diagnosis of a hydatidiform mole is made by ultrasound scanning. Suction evacuation is performed and the diagnosis of a complete hydatidiform mole is confirmed by histological examination of the curettings.

   What is the most appropriate next step in the management?

   A. Give intramuscular methotrexate daily for five days.
   B. Perform a hysterectomy.
   C. Perform a repeat suction evacuation after 2 weeks.
   D. Perform serum beta hCG levels weekly till the test becomes negative.
   E. Perform urine hCG weekly till the test becomes negative.

4. A 42-year-old woman in her fifth pregnancy complains of excessive vomiting and mild vaginal bleeding for two weeks at a POA of 10 weeks. The fundal height corresponds to 18 weeks. Ultrasound scan demonstrates a snowstorm appearance in the uterus and bilateral theca-lutein cysts.

   What is the best management option?

   A. Perform a hysterectomy.
   B. Perform a hysterotomy and bilateral ovarian cystectomy.
   C. Perform suction evacuation.
   D. Perform medical evacuation with an oxytocin infusion.
   E. Perform suction evacuation after ripening the cervix with prostaglandin.

5. A woman complains of excessive vomiting and mild vaginal bleeding for two weeks at a POA of 12 weeks. The fundal height corresponds to 16 weeks. The

cervical os is closed. Ultrasound scan demonstrates a snowstorm appearance in part of the uterus together with a foetus. The crown-rump length corresponds to 10 weeks. The foetal heart beat is absent. What is the best management option?

A. Carry out medical termination with vaginal misoprostol.

B. Carry out medical termination with an oxytocin infusion.

C. Perform suction evacuation.

D. Perform a total abdominal hysterectomy.

E. Perform suction evacuation after giving oral mifepristone.

6. A 30-year-old woman with one child underwent suction evacuation of a complete hydatidiform mole, which was confirmed by histology. Her serum beta hCG level is 20000 IU/L 8 weeks after evacuation.
   What is the most appropriate management?

   A. Commence treatment with combination chemotherapy.

B. Commence treatment with intramuscular methotrexate.

C. Perform a hysterectomy.

D. Perform repeat suction evacuation.

E. Repeat the serum beta hCG test after 4 weeks.

7. A 40-year-old woman complains of irregular bleeding for 7 months after delivery of her fourth baby. Curettage is performed and histology reveals a choriocarcinoma. Her serum beta hCG level is 2×10^5 IU/L.

   What is the most appropriate next step in the management?

   A. Commence treatment with intramuscular methotrexate.

   B. Commence treatment with multi-agent combination chemotherapy.

   C. Perform a hysterectomy.

   D. Perform a repeat evacuation after 2 weeks.

   E. Repeat serum hCG after 4 weeks.

ANSWERS AND EXPLANATIONS

Q. 1 (D)

Q. 2 (C)

Explanation for questions 1 and 2

Occurrence of a hydatidiform mole can be suspected as she has a POA followed by vaginal bleeding and excessive vomiting. The clinical diagnosis of a complete hydatidiform mole is confirmed by the presence of a snowstorm appearance without foetal parts in the ultrasound scan. The diagnosis can be suspected if the serum β-hCG is inappropriately high for the POA. Serial serum β hCG tests are not indicated.

The best management option for a hydatidiform mole is suction evacuation, as the negative pressure prevents trophoblastic embolization. Cervical preparation with

misoprostol or prostaglandin should be avoided to prevent trophoblastic embolization. Oxytocin should not be commenced till the evacuation is complete. Hysterectomy is the treatment of choice for women over the age of 40 years, especially if there are other risk factors such as large theca-lutein cysts, significant uterine enlargement, or pre-treatment hCG level more than 10^5.

Q. 3 (D)

After histological confirmation of a molar pregnancy hCG levels are estimated once a week, until the levels return to normal. If the hCG levels return to normal within 56 days after evacuation, hCG levels will be checked monthly for 6 months from the day of evacuation. If the hCG levels return to normal more than 56 days after evacuation, hCG levels will be checked monthly for 6 months, after the values become normal. Urine hCG test is not useful as quantitative estimation is not possible. Routine second uterine evacuation is not recommended. If symptoms persist, serum hCG levels and ultrasound scanning should be done. Hysterectomy is recommended for women over the age of 40 years, especially if there are other risk factors, such as large theca-lutein cysts, significant uterine enlargement, or pre-treatment hCG level more than 10^5.

Q. 4 (A)

Hysterectomy is the treatment of choice for this woman as she is a multipara over the age of 40 years, and there are other risk factors for occurrence of choriocarcinoma, such as large theca-lutein cysts and significant uterine enlargement.

Q. 5 (C)

Suction evacuation is the method of choice, for evacuation of a partial molar pregnancy, except when the size of the foetus precludes the procedure. Since the CRL corresponds to 10 weeks, suction evacuation is the best treatment option for this woman. Medical evacuation is recommended if the foetus is larger than 12 weeks. However, there is an increased risk of persistent trophoblastic disease.

Q. 6 (B)

Since this woman has a high serum hCG level 8 weeks after suction evacuation, she is at risk of developing gestational trophoblastic neoplasia. Therefore, the most appropriate management is to commence chemotherapy. Since this patient is under 40 years of age and the antecedent pregnancy is a molar pregnancy which was evacuated 8 weeks ago, she has a low risk according to the FIGO scoring system. Therefore, she can be commenced on single agent chemotherapy, with methotrexate and leucovorin rescue. Methotrexate 50 mg intramuscularly (or 1 mg/kg) is given every other day for 4 days, with leucovorin 15 mg (or 0.1 mg/kg) 24–30 hours after each dose of methotrexate. The course is repeated after 6 rest days till the serum hCG becomes negative. Treatment is continued for 6 consecutive weeks after the hCG becomes negative. Combination chemotherapy is not necessary as the score is less than 6. Chemotherapy is the most important mode of treatment for choriocarcinoma.

Q. 7 (B)

This woman is at high risk as she has a prognostic score of 7:
- Antecedent normal pregnancy—2
- Age more than 40—1
- Antecedent pregnancy 7 months ago—2
- Serum hCG level 2×10^5—2

Therefore, she needs treatment with multi-agent combination chemotherapy with EMA-CO. EMA-CO is etoposide, methotrexate with leucovorin rescue and actinomycin D, given on day 1 and 2 and cyclophosphamide and vincristine (Oncovin) given on day 8.

Day 1: Etoposide 100 mg/m² by infusion in 200 ml of normal saline (NS) over 30 min. Actinomycin D (Act D) 0.5 mg IV and methotrexate 100 mg/m² IV or 200 mg/m² by infusion over 12 hours.

Day 2: Etoposide 100 mg/m² by infusion in 200 ml NS over 30 min, ActD 0.5 mg IV. Leucovorin 15 mg 12 hourly × 4 doses IM or orally beginning 24 hrs after starting methotrexate.

Day 8: Cyclophosphamide 600 mg/m² by infusion in NS over 30 min Vincristine 1 mg/m² IV

REFERENCES

- Gestational Trophoblastic Disease (RCOG Green-top Guideline No. 38): Published: 04/03/2010.
- RANZCOG Statement for the management of gestational trophoblastic disease, C-Gyn 31, November 2013.

14

Menopause and Hormone Replacement Therapy

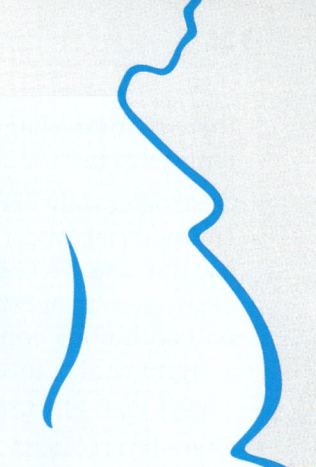

DIAGNOSIS

Menopause is diagnosed by the absence of menstrual periods for one year, in an otherwise healthy woman over the age of 45 years, who is not on hormonal treatment. The diagnosis is based on symptoms in a woman who has undergone a hysterectomy.

FSH levels are used to diagnose menopause in women aged between 40 and 45 years, who have vasomotor symptoms and irregular periods.

Premature ovarian failure is diagnosed in women less than 40 years of age by menopausal symptoms, absent or infrequent periods and elevated FSH levels on 2 blood samples taken 4–6 weeks apart.

Do not use anti-müllerian hormone, inhibin A, inhibin B, oestradiol, antral follicle count or ovarian volume to diagnose menopause in women over the age of 45 years.

Indications for HRT

- Relief of vasomotor and other menopausal symptoms (short-term).
- Prevention/treatment of osteoporosis (long-term).

Treatment is most beneficial if commenced before the age of 60 years or within 10 years of menopause.

The dose should be reduced when treatment is commenced in women over the age of 60 years.

The diet and lifestyle should be optimized.

CONTRAINDICATIONS

Absolute Contraindications

- Undiagnosed abnormal vaginal bleeding.
- Active thromboembolic disorder.
- Acute-phase myocardial infarction.
- Previous stroke.
- Suspected or active breast or endometrial carcinoma.
- Active liver disease with abnormal liver function tests.
- Porphyria cutanea tarda.

Relative Contraindications

- Past history of benign breast disease.
- Presence of fibroids.
- Chronic stable liver disease.
- Migraine.

COMPLICATIONS AND RISKS

Increased Risk of Cancer

- Increased risk of breast cancer occurs with long-term treatment with combined HRT (>5 years). Any increase in the risk of breast cancer is related to treatment duration and reduces after stopping HRT. Risk is much less with oestrogen-only HRT but increases after 10 years of treatment.
- According to the WHO trial there is no increased risk of ovarian cancer. However,

there may be a slightly increased risk after long-term use for about 8 or more years.

- Oestrogen only HRT increases the risk of endometrial cancer, but this can be avoided by the use of combined or sequential oestrogen/progestogen therapy. Women on continuous combined regimens are at a significantly lower risk of endometrial cancer than untreated women.

- There is a reduced risk of colorectal cancer with the use of oral combined HRT.

- There is no increased risk of cervical cancer in women who are on HRT.

- HRT is not contraindicated in women who have been treated for squamous cell carcinoma or adenocarcinoma of the cervix.

Risk of Cardiovascular Disease

- HRT is associated with an increased risk of stroke, especially in women over the age of 60 years.

- HRT should not be given to women who have, or are at risk of cardiovascular disease, unless if treatment is essential.

- Oestrogen only HRT is associated with no or reduced risk of coronary heart disease.

- Combined oestrogen and progestogen HRT cause a little or no increase in the risk of coronary heart disease, in women who are within 10 years of menopause.

- There is an increased risk of venous thromboembolism, especially in women with other risk factors. The risk is less with transdermal HRT.

Type 2 Diabetes

- The risk of developing type 2 diabetes is not increased by HRT.

- HRT has no adverse effects on the blood sugar control in those with diabetes.

It is necessary to perform the following investigations before commencing HRT to exclude risk factors.

- ECG, lipid profile and fasting blood sugar
- Echocardiograph and assessment by a cardiologist if coronary heart disease is suspected.
- Liver function tests.
- Mammogram.
- Cervical smear.
- Transvaginal and abdominal ultrasound scan.

TREATMENT OPTIONS

Hormonal Treatment Options

- Oestrogen should be given continuously. The oestrogen commonly used is oestradiol. The dose can range from 50 mcg– 2 mg. Prempak C has 625 mcg–1.25 mg of conjugated oestrogen while premarin (oestrogen only) has 300 mcg, 625 mcg and 1.25 mg tablets.

- Progestogen is given in addition to oestrogen in women who have an intact uterus, to reduce the risk of endometrial hyperplasia. Norethisterone 700 mcg–1 mg, medroxyprogesterone 2.5–10 mg, levonorgestrel 7 mcg–10 mcg, norgestrel 150 mcg and dydrogesterone 10 mg are the commonly used progestogens.

- **A levonorgestrel-releasing intrauterine system** (LNG IUS) can be inserted to protect the endometrium in women receiving oestrogen therapy. Systemic side effects are less though the impact on the risk of breast cancer remains unclear.

- Oral treatment is the first preference.

- A sequential combined regimen is recommended for women who have reached menopause within one year of commencing HRT. Oestrogen is given continuously and progestogen is given for 12–14 days per month. This will result in monthly withdrawal bleeding. Sequential combined regimen is more protective for the breast than continuous combined treatment.

- Continuous combined therapies offer 'period free' therapy for patients who are

≥ 54 years, or more than 1 year post-menopausal at any age.

- Always commence with low dose preparations.
- Transdermal patches are used to avoid the first pass effect through the liver and are recommended for those at increased risk of thromboembolism.
- Low dose vaginal oestrogen creams can be used for those with urogenital atrophy.

Non-hormonal Treatment Options

- Paroxetine and fluoxetine which are selective serotonin re-uptake inhibitor (SSRI) antidepressants, can be used to relieve vasomotor symptoms, in women with breast cancer who are not taking tamoxifen.

- Selective noradrenaline reuptake inhibitor (SNRI) venlafaxine 37.5 mg twice daily can be used in those with breast cancer.
- Both these groups of drugs have a high incidence of nausea. They also cause loss of libido.
- Clonidine, a centrally active alpha-2 agonist, is found to have some effects in reducing vasomotor symptoms.
- Anti-epileptic drug gabapentin should only be offered to treat hot flushes in women with breast cancer, but causes drowsiness dizziness and fatigue.
- Didronel, alendronate, clodronate, pamidronate, and residronate are bisphosphonates which inhibit bone absorption and normalize bone turnover.

QUESTIONS

1. **A 43-year-old woman who had a total abdominal hysterectomy and bilateral salpingo-oophorectomy for endometriosis attends the clinic after 1 year with vasomotor symptoms.**

   What is the best management option?

   A. Continuous combined hormone replacement therapy.

   B. Oestrogen only hormone replacement therapy.

   C. Raloxifene.

   D. Sequential combined hormone replacement therapy.

   E. Tibalone.

2. **A 50-year-old otherwise healthy woman complains of vasomotor symptoms. She has a period of amenorrhoea of 3 months.**

   What is the best hormonal replacement therapy for this woman?

   A. Continuous combined hormone replacement therapy.

   B. Oestrogen only hormone replacement therapy.

   C. Raloxifene.

   D. Sequential combined hormone replacement therapy.

   E. Tibalone.

3. **A 55-year-old otherwise healthy woman complains of severe hot flashes. She has reached menopause 3 years ago.**

   What is the best hormonal replacement therapy for this patient?

   A. Continuous combined hormone replacement therapy.

   B. Oestrogen only hormone replacement therapy.

   C. Raloxifene.

   D. Sequential combined hormone replacement therapy.

   E. Tibalone.

4. **A 55-year-old woman, who was successfully treated for breast cancer 3 years ago and is on tamoxifen, complains of severe backache due to osteoporosis. She does not have vasomotor symptoms.**

   What is the best treatment option?

A. Fluoxetine.

B. Oestrogen only hormone replacement therapy.

C. Raloxifene.

D. Sequential combined hormone replacement therapy.

E. Venlafaxine.

5. **A 55-year-old woman, who was successfully treated for breast cancer 3 years ago, complains of severe hot flashes. She is on tamoxifen.**

   What is the best treatment option?

   A. Fluoxetine.

   B. Oestrogen only hormone replacement therapy.

   C. Raloxifene.

   D. Sequential combined hormone replacement therapy.

   E. Venlafaxine.

6. **A 39-year-old woman who has had amenorrhoea for 1 year complains of hot flashes.**

   Which of the following is the best method to diagnose the occurrence of menopause in this patient?

A. Perform FSH level on one occasion.

B. Perform FSH level twice within 4–6 weeks.

C. Perform anti-müllerian hormone level.

D. Perform inhibin A level.

E. Perform oestradiol level.

7. **A 39-year-old woman who has had amenorrhoea for 1 year complains of hot flashes and irritability. Her last child is 3 years of age. Occurrence of menopause is diagnosed by the presence of high FSH levels on two occasions 6 weeks apart.**

   What is the best treatment option?

   A. Combined oral contraceptive pills.

   B. Continuous combined hormone replacement therapy.

   C. Fluoxetine.

   D. Oestrogen only hormone replacement therapy.

   E. Sequential combined hormone replacement therapy.

ANSWERS AND EXPLANATIONS

Q. 1 (B)

Oestrogen only hormone replacement therapy carry a reduced risk of breast cancer, but an increased risk of endometrial hyperplasia and endometrial cancer. Therefore, it is recommended for women who have undergone a hysterectomy for a benign condition. There is an increased risk of breast cancer with long-term treatment with combined HRT (>5 years). The increased risk is related to treatment duration. As this patient is 43 years of age, she will need long-term treatment. Therefore, the best treatment option for this woman is oestrogen only HRT.

Q. 2 (D)

Since the last menstrual period has occurred less than one year ago commencing

sequential combined HRT is the best option. Oestrogen is given continuously and progestogen is given for 12–14 days per month. This will result in monthly withdrawal bleeding and is more protective for the breast than continuous combined treatment. Continuous combined therapy can be offered after 1 year if she prefers to avoid withdrawal bleeding. Oestrogen only HRT carry a high risk of endometrial cancer and is not recommended for a woman with a uterus. Raloxifene does not relieve vasomotor symptoms.

Q. 3 (A)

Continuous combined HRT is the best option for this patient as she is more than 54 years of age and has reached menopause more than 1 year ago.

Q. 4 (C)

Raloxifene is a selective oestrogen receptor modulator. They are specific and do not engage the oestrogen receptors in all tissues, but do so selectively. They exert protective oestrogen action on the skeleton, but avoid adverse effects on the breast and the endometrium. Therefore, raloxifene can be used to prevent further bone loss in this patient.

Q. 5 (E)

Selective noradrenaline reuptake inhibitor (SNRI) venlafaxine 37.5 mg twice daily can be used in those with breast cancer, as oestrogen containing HRT is contraindicated. Venlafaxine will reduce hot flashes, but has no effect on preventing osteoporosis. The mechanism of action is not clear, but the antidepressant action may play a role. However, hot flashes are relieved within one week, but the antidepressant action takes several weeks. An imbalance in serotonin can cause hot flashes. The most common adverse effects are insomnia, nausea, constipation, and anorexia. A dose of 37.5 mg is effective but can be increased to 70 mg. An enzyme called CYP2D6 helps tamoxifen work in the body. Fluoxetine and paroxetine can interfere with how CYP2D6 works and might reduce the effectiveness of tamoxifen against breast cancer. Therefore, these drugs are best avoided in those on tamoxifen.

Q. 6 (B)

Premature ovarian failure is diagnosed in women aged less than 40 years, by menopausal symptoms, absent or infrequent periods and elevated FSH levels on 2 blood samples taken 4–6 weeks apart.

Q. 7 (E)

Sequential combined therapy is the best as she needs long-term therapy and sequential therapy is more protective to the breast and stimulates monthly menstruation.

REFERENCE

- Menopause: Diagnosis and Management, NICE guidelines [NG23], Published date: November 2015.

15

Endometriosis

Endometriosis is defined as the presence of endometrial surface epithelium and/or the presence of endometrial glands and stroma outside the lining of the uterine cavity.

These ectopic endometrial tissues respond in varying degrees to the cyclical changes in ovarian hormones and during menstruation bleeding occurs from the endometriotic deposits. This produces a local inflammatory reaction. Subsequent fibrosis will cause formation of adhesions between organs. Bleeding into ovarian implants will result in formation of chocolate cysts or endometriomas.

SYMPTOMS

- Symptoms will depend on the site and extent of the lesion.
- The disease may be symptomless and may be a coincidental finding during surgery or during investigation of a patient complaining of infertility.
- Symptoms are mostly related to the genital tract. Other organs are rarely affected.

Female Reproductive Tract

- Dysmenorrhoea
- Lower abdominal and pelvic pain
- Dyspareunia
- Low back pain

- Infertility
- Short menstrual cycles

Urinary Tract

- Cyclical haematuria/ dysuria
- Ureteric obstruction

Gastrointestinal Tract

- Dyschezia
- Cyclical rectal bleeding
- Obstruction

Surgical Scars/Umbilicus

- Cyclical pain and bleeding

Lung

- Cyclical haemoptysis
- Haemopneumothorax

EXAMINATION FINDINGS

- Endometriotic nodules are most reliably detected, when clinical examination is performed during menstruation.
- Pelvic tenderness, a fixed retroverted uterus, tender uterosacral ligaments, or enlarged ovaries/ovarian masses are suggestive of endometriosis.
- Palpation of deeply infiltrating nodules on the uterosacral ligaments, or in the pouch of Douglas, or presence of visible lesions in the vagina, or on the cervix makes the diagnosis more certain.

- Diagnosis should be considered in women with symptoms even if the clinical examination is normal.
- Chronic pelvic inflammatory disease should be considered in the differential diagnosis. Both conditions cause chronic pelvic pain, dysmenorrhoea, dyspareunia, short menstrual cycles and infertility.

INVESTIGATIONS

- Transvaginal ultrasound scan is the first step in the diagnosis. Ultrasound appearance of an ovarian endometrioma includes ground glass echogenicity, one to four compartments and no papillary structures with detectable blood flow. TVUS is also used to diagnose recto-vaginal endometriosis.
- Ca 125 is mildly elevated but is not used in the diagnosis.
- Laparoscopy is the gold standard in the diagnosis. Laparoscopy allows direct visualization and biopsy. Histological examination should be performed. The diagnosis should be confirmed whenever possible by positive histology. However, the diagnosis cannot be excluded by negative histology. Visual inspection is usually adequate but histological confirmation of at least one lesion is ideal. Histology is necessary to exclude malignancy in deeply infiltrating disease and in ovarian endometriomas.

TREATMENT

Symptomless deposits detected at laparoscopy do not require treatment.

Analgesics

NSAIDs are used to treat pelvic pain and dysmenorrhoea.

Hormonal Treatment

Hormonal treatment with long-term ovarian suppression is the mainstay of treatment, in those who do not need immediate fertility.

Surgical management can be superimposed if required.

Treatment must be continued for 3–6 months.

- Combined oral contraceptive pills
  - Can be used cyclically but continuous treatment is preferred.
  - Is recommended for mild cases.
- Progestogens
  - Oral medroxyprogesterone acetate 10–30 mg daily for 3–6 months.
  - Depot medroxyprogesterone acetate injections, 150 mg IM once a month for 3–6 months, is the preferred progestogen.
  - Insertion of a levonorgestrel releasing intrauterine device.
- Letrozole
  - Inhibits aromatase activity within the endometriotic lesions, thereby reducing the formation of oestrogens.
  - The dose is 5 mg administered daily for 3 months.
  - Osteoporosis and other effects of oestrogen deprivation can occur with long-term therapy.
- Danazol
  - 400–800 mg daily for 3–6 months
- GnRH analogues
  - These are administered intramuscularly in a dose of 3.75 mg once a month (the dose can be variable) for 3–6 months with add back therapy.
  - Not recommended for adolescents as they may not have reached the maximum bone density.

Surgery

- Is the mainstay of therapy in infertile patients.
- Surgery is performed by laparoscopy. Following surgical options can be carried out.

– Diathermy ablation of endometriotic deposits.

– Adhesiolysis.

– Cystectomy is the best option for endometriotic cysts.

– Drainage and diathermy of cysts is not recommended as recurrence is common.

• Postoperative medical treatment may be given to prevent recurrence, but is better avoided in infertile patients as ovulation will be impaired.

• Hysterectomy and BSO is the definitive treatment. HRT is postponed for 1 year to prevent recurrence.

ADENOMYOSIS

Adenomyosis is a condition in which endometrial glands and stroma are present within the uterine musculature. The ectopic endometrial tissue appears to induce hypertrophy and hyperplasia of the surrounding myometrium, which result in a smooth uniformly enlarged uterus, similar to the enlargement of the pregnant uterus. However, the uterus will be firm in consistency in adenomyosis while it will be soft in pregnancy. A single interstitial or submucous fibroid can cause a similar enlargement. Sometimes adenomyosis causes small diffuse deposits which can only be seen by microscopy. Occasionally adenomyosis forms nodules (termed adenomyomas), which clinically resemble leiomyomas. The uterus generally does not exceed the size of a pregnant uterus at 12–14 weeks of gestation.

Adenomyosis usually occurs in multiparous women between 40 and 50 years of age. Previous uterine surgery, genetic factors and smoking may predispose to its occurrence.

Symptoms

• Heavy menstrual bleeding
• Dysmenorrhoea

• Dyspareunia
• Chronic abdominal, back and pelvic pain

Signs

Smooth tender firm enlargement of the uterus which is usually not larger than 12–14 weeks in size.

Differential Diagnosis—Uterine Fibroids

A single submucous or an interstitial fibroid can cause a similar enlargement, but usually fibroids cause irregular uterine enlargement which can reach a larger size.

DIAGNOSIS

• Transvaginal ultrasound scanning

  – Globular smooth enlargement of the uterus with uniform myometrial thickening

  – Endometrial/myometrial interphase becomes less clear

  – Presence of myometrial cysts

• MRI scanning

However, the diagnosis can be confirmed only by histological examination of the uterus removed at hysterectomy.

TREATMENT

• NSAIDs for pelvic pain and dysmenorrhoea.

• Tranexamic acid and mefenamic acid can be given during menstruation to reduce the flow.

• Hormonal treatment can be tried as in the case of endometriosis, but the results are poor.

• Endometrial ablation and uterine artery embolization are options.

• The only definitive treatment is hysterectomy.

QUESTIONS

1. A 29-year-old woman complains of infertility for two years with dysmenorrhoea and deep dyspareunia. Bimanual vaginal examination reveals a retroverted uterus with limited mobility and tenderness in the pouch of Douglas.

   What is the next step in the management?

   A. Perform a diagnostic laparoscopy.

   B. Perform a hysterosalpingogram.

   C. Perform a laparotomy.

   D. Perform a transvaginal ultrasound scan.

   E. Treat with GnRH analogues.

2. A 29-year-old woman complains of infertility for two years with dysmenorrhoea and deep dyspareunia. Bimanual vaginal examination reveals a retroverted uterus with limited mobility and tenderness in the pouch of Douglas. Transvaginal scan is normal. She wishes to conceive soon.

   What is the next step in the management?

   A. Perform a laparoscopy.

   B. Perform a hysterosalpingogram.

   C. Perform a laparotomy.

   D. Treat with GnRH analogues.

   E. Treat with medroxyprogesterone acetate injections.

3. A 33-year-old woman complains of infertility for three years with dysmenorrhea and deep dyspareunia. Laparoscopy reveals endometriotic deposits in the pouch of Douglas, peritubal adhesions and an interstitial fibroid measuring about 6 × 5 cm. Both tubes are patent. She wishes to conceive soon.

   What is the most appropriate management?

   A. Perform diathermy cauterization of the deposits, adhesiolysis and myomectomy through the laparoscope.

   B. Perform tubal reconstruction, diathermy cauterization of the deposits and myomectomy through a laparotomy.

   C. Treat with combined oral contraceptive pills continuously.

   D. Treat with GnRH analogues.

   E. Treat with medroxyprogesterone acetate injections.

4. A 38-year-old woman who has two children complains of dysmenorrhea and dyspareunia. Transvaginal ultrasound scan shows a thin walled cyst 4 × 4 cm in diameter with echogenic fluid and no solid areas in the right ovary. She has no fertility wishes.

   What is the first line treatment option?

   A. Perform laparoscopic cystectomy.

   B. Treat with combined oral contraceptive pills continuously.

   C. Treat with GnRH analogues.

   D. Treat with medroxyprogesterone acetate injections.

   E. Treat with oral danazol.

5. A 30-year-old infertile woman complains of dysmenorrhea and dyspareunia. Transvaginal ultrasound scan shows a thin walled cyst 4 × 4 cm in diameter with echogenic fluid and no solid areas in the right ovary. She wishes to conceive soon.

   What is the best treatment option?

   A. Perform laparoscopic cystectomy.

   B. Treat with combined oral contraceptive pills continuously.

   C. Treat with GnRH analogues.

   D. Treat with medroxyprogesterone acetate injections.

   E. Treat with oral danazol.

6. A 44-year-old woman with one child, 5 years of age complains of chronic pelvic pain, severe dysmenorrhea which outlasts the period and dyspareunia for three years. Transvaginal ultrasound scan shows a thin walled cyst 7 cm ×

7 cm in diameter with echogenic fluid and no solid areas in the right ovary. Laparoscopic cystectomy has been performed for a similar endometriotic cyst when she was treated for infertility 6 years ago.

What is the best treatment option?

A. Perform hysterectomy and bilateral salpingo-oophorectomy.
B. Perform laparoscopic cystectomy.
C. Treat with combined oral contraceptive pills continuously.
D. Treat with GnRH analogues.
E. Treat with medroxyprogesterone acetate injections.

ANSWERS AND EXPLANATIONS

Q. 1 (D)

Q. 2 (A)

Q. 3 (A)

Explanation for questions 1, 2 and 3

Since this woman is infertile and has dysmenorrhea, dyspareunia and frequent periods, she is most probably having endometriosis. The first step is to perform a transvaginal scan, which will show endometriotic cysts and nodules. However, small endometriotic deposits and peritubal adhesions may not be visible on the scan. Therefore, if the scan is negative the next step in the management is to perform a laparoscopy for diagnosis and treatment.

The most appropriate treatment is laparoscopy, diathermy cauterization of the deposits, myomectomy and adhesiolysis. Medical treatment will result in infertility during treatment and in some cases for several months after stopping treatment (such as in the case of DMPA injections).

Q. 4 (D)

Q. 5 (A)

Explanation for questions 4 and 5

Since she has symptoms of endometriosis and the cyst has thin walls, with echogenic fluid and no solid areas, it is most probably an endometriotic cyst. As the cyst is smaller than 5 cm and the woman does not desire fertility (Q4), medical treatment can be tried first. Both GnRH analogues and DMPA are equally effective, but DMPA is the first line treatment in Sri Lanka and other developing countries because of the lower cost.

If the woman desires fertility (Q5), the most appropriate treatment is laparoscopic cystectomy, diathermy cauterisation of other deposits and adhesiolysis. Medical treatment will result in infertility during treatment and in some cases for several months after stopping treatment (such as in the case of DMPA injections).

Q. 6 (A)

Since this woman is 44 years of age, has severe symptoms which have recurred after previous conservative surgery, TAH and BSO is the best treatment option, as pelvic endometriotic deposits will burn out once the ovaries are removed. HRT is commenced only after 1 year to allow time for healing of endometriotic deposits. If HRT is commenced before healing, these can become active again due to presence of oestrogen and progesterone.

REFERENCES

- Guideline of the European Society of Human Reproduction and Embryology—ESHRE Endometriosis Guideline Development Group—September 2013.
- Endometriosis, Investigation and Management (Green-top Guideline No. 24), Published: 01/10/2006.

16

Endometrial Carcinoma

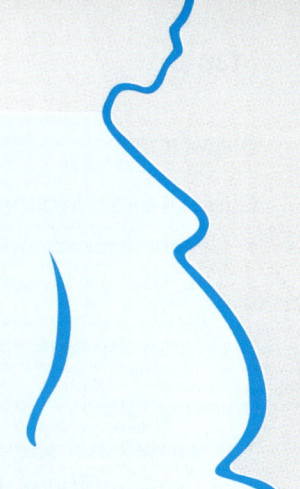

AETIOLOGY

The main aetiological factor is increase in the oestrogen levels. After menopause majority of the oestrogen entering the circulation is produced by aromatization of peripheral androgens mainly in the adipose tissue. Circulating oestrogen levels are increased in postmenopausal women with diabetes.

- Obesity.
  - Body fat produces oestrogen, and women with excess fat have a higher level of oestrogen than women without excess fat. The higher level of oestrogen is believed to increase the risk of cancer.
- Nulliparity.
- Early puberty before 12 years and late menopause after 52 years.
  - Early puberty and late menopause increase the number of years that the endometrium is exposed to oestrogen.
- Oestrogen replacement therapy with unopposed oestrogen without added progesterone.
- Endometrial hyperplasia especially atypical hyperplasia.
- Diabetes mellitus.
- Hypertension.
- Polycystic ovarian syndrome due to high level of oestrogen.
- Treatment with tamoxifen.

- Other cancers.
  - Cancers of the breast, ovary, and colon are linked with an increased risk of endometrial cancer.
- Family history.
- Functioning ovarian tumours.
- Pelvic irradiation.
- Gall bladder disease.

PROTECTIVE FACTORS

Smoking and progesterone

Smoking is protective because it changes the metabolism of oestrogen and cause weight loss and early menopause. This effect lasts for a long time after smoking is stopped.

Progesterone reduces risk of endometrial cancer by 30–50% over 10–20 years.

Grand multiparity is also a protective factor.

CLINICAL PRESENTATION

- Usually early diagnosis is possible because of early occurrence of abnormal uterine bleeding or postmenopausal bleeding.
- The commonest presentation is post-menopausal bleeding.
- Postmenopausal discharge, particularly a blood stained discharge may be the presenting symptom.
- Perimenopausal women will present with intermenstrual bleeding or with heavy periods only.

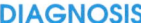

DIAGNOSIS

Clinical Examination

- Cervix appears normal
- The uterus is usually normal in size or slightly bulky. Uterine enlargement occurs only in the later stages.

Investigations

- Transvaginal scanning
  - An endometrial thickness of more than 4 mm in postmenopausal women, or more than 10 mm in premenopausal women, is suspicious of endometrial carcinoma and requires further investigations. Focal endometrial thickening is especially significant. An endometrial thickness of less than 4 mm has a negative predictive value.
- Confirmation of diagnosis is by histology
  - Pipelle sampling can be done as an outpatient procedure and is used in premenopausal patients with uniform endometrial thickening. It is not suitable for postmenopausal patients because the endometrium is thin and the incidence of malignancy is high.
  - Dilatation and curettage and fractional curettage are of limited value, because a small initial lesion can be missed.
  - Hysteroscopy and directed biopsy is the gold standard of arriving at a histological diagnosis and is essential if there is focal endometrial thickening.

The FIGO cancer staging system for staging of endometrial carcinoma

Stage	
I	Tumour confined to the corpus uteri
IA	Less than 50% invasion of the myometrium
IB	More than 50% invasion of the myometrium.
II	Tumour invades cervical stroma but does not extend beyond the uterus

Contd.

Contd.

III	Local and/or regional spread of the tumour
IIIA	Tumour invades serosa of the corpus uteri and/or adnexae.
IIIB	Vaginal and/or parametrial involvement
IIIC1	Positive pelvic lymph nodes
IIIC2	Positive para-aortic lymph nodes with or without pelvic nodes
IV	Tumour invades bladder/bowel mucosa, and/or distant metastases
IVA	Tumour invasion of bladder and/or bowel mucosa
IVB	Distant metastases including intra-abdominal and/or inguinal lymph nodes

Histopathological Grades (G)

- Gx—Grade cannot be assessed;
- G1—Well differentiated;
- G2—Moderately differentiated;
- G3—Poorly differentiated or undifferentiated.

Pathology

- The commonest subtype is endometrioid carcinoma. Histology resembles the normal endometrium, but the architecture is much more complicated.
- An adenoacanthoma or an adenosquamous carcinoma occurs when squamous metaplasia occur within an adenocarcinoma.
- Papillary, serous and clear cell carcinomas are aggressive forms of endometrial carcinoma, and primary squamous cell carcinoma is a rare variant.

Adverse Prognostic Factors

- Tumour grade 3 (poorly differentiated)
- Deep myometrial invasion (FIGO stage IB)
- Lymphovascular channel involvement
- Positive peritoneal cytology
- Serous or papillary tumours
- Clear cell tumours
- Cervical involvement (stage II)

Low risk: Endometrioid type
                   histology
                   Stage IA (G1 and G2)

Intermediate risk: Endometrioid type
                   histology
                   Stage IA G3
                   Stage IB (G1 and G2)

High risk: Stage IB G3 and above
                   with endometrioid type
                   histology

All stages with non-endometrioid type histology.

TREATMENT

Surgery

- It is preferable to perform a MRI scan prior to surgery to determine the extent of myometrial invasion and involvement of lymph nodes.

- Surgery is the treatment of choice for endometrial carcinoma.

- For low risk patients with stage IA, G1–G2 endometriod tumours the treatment of choice is total abdominal hysterectomy and bilateral salpingo-oophorectomy. Peritoneal washings are taken, lymph nodes are palpated and suspicious nodes are sampled.

- If higher risk features are found at surgery or on histopathological examination, adjuvant radiotherapy may be considered in conjunction with an oncologist.

- Total abdominal hysterectomy, BSO, pelvic and para-aortic lymphadenectomy and peritoneal washings for cytology, is the standard treatment for women with the following risk factors

  - G3 tumours

  - Papillary, serous or clear cell types

  - Greater than 50% myometrial invasion (Stage IB)

  - Suspicion of nodal involvement on CT or MRI scan

- Stage 2 cancers are treated with radical hysterectomy, BSO, pelvic and para-aortic lymphadenectomy.

- Maximum debulking is indicated in stage III and IV tumours.

- Only palliative surgery may be possible in stage IV B cases.

RADIOTHERAPY (RT)

Stage IA (G1–G2)	Observation without adjuvant therapy
Stage IA G3	Observation or vaginal BT. If adverse prognostic factors are present pelvic RT and/or adjunctive chemotherapy could be considered.
Stage IB (G1 –G2)	Observation or vaginal BT. If adverse prognostic factors are present pelvic RT and/or chemotherapy could be considered.
Stage IB G3	Pelvic RT If negative prognostic factors are present combination of radiation and chemotherapy could be considered
Stage II	Pelvic RT and vaginal BT
Stage III–IV	Chemotherapy and sequential radiotherapy

- Radiotherapy is not indicated for G1 tumours without serosal involvement, and G2 tumours with less than 50% myometrial invasion.

- Radiotherapy is of uncertain benefit even in higher risk women without extra uterine disease.

- Adjuvant radiotherapy is indicated for the very high risk cases such as G3 tumours, greater than 50% myometrial invasion or positive lymph node involvement.

- External beam radiotherapy is indicated for pelvic recurrence.

- Vaginal brachytherapy (BT) is advisable to prevent vaginal recurrence and in the presence of cervical involvement.

- Vaginal brachytherapy and external beam radiation were found to be equally effective in intermediate risk patients but the quality of life was better in patients who received vaginal brachytherapy.

CHEMOTHERAPY

Adjuvant chemotherapy consists of combination of taxanes, doxorubicin and platins (particularly cisplatin and carboplatin). Adjuvant chemotherapy has been found to increase survival in stages III and IV cancer more than added radiotherapy.

Hormonal Therapy

Hormonal therapy is only beneficial in certain types of endometrial cancer with a large number of progesterone receptors.

Follow Up

All patients should receive more frequent pelvic examinations and ultrasound scanning for 5 years following treatment. Examinations conducted every 3–4 months are recommended for the first two years following treatment, and every 6 months for the next 3 years.

QUESTIONS

1. A 50-year-old woman who had reached menopause 2 years ago presents with a single episode of postmenopausal bleeding. Abdominal and vaginal examinations are normal. Transvaginal scan reveals an endometrial thickness of 3 mm.

    What is the most appropriate next step in the management?

    A. Perform fractional curettage.

    B. Perform hysteroscopy and biopsy.

    C. Perform pipelle aspiration.

    D. Perform total hysterectomy.

    E. Review in 3 months or earlier if bleeding recurs.

2. A 51-year-old woman who had reached menopause 1 year ago presents with a single episode of a few drops of post-menopausal bleeding. Abdominal and vaginal examinations are normal. Trans-vaginal scan reveals uniform endometrial thickness of 6 mm.

    What is the most suitable next step in the management?

    A. Perform fractional curettage.

    B. Perform hysteroscopy and biopsy.

    C. Perform pipelle aspiration.

D. Perform total hysterectomy.

E. Review in 3 months or earlier if bleeding recurs.

3. A 54-year-old woman who had reached menopause 3 years ago presents with a single episode of postmenopausal bleeding. Abdominal and vaginal examinations are normal. Transvaginal scan reveals an endometrial thickness of 4 mm with an area of focal thickening of 8 mm.

    What is the most appropriate next step in the management?

    A. Perform fractional curettage.

    B. Perform hysteroscopy and biopsy.

    C. Perform pipelle aspiration.

    D. Perform a total hysterectomy.

    E. Review in 3 months or earlier if bleeding recurs.

4. A 65-year-old woman presents with postmenopausal bleeding. Hysteroscopy, biopsy and histology reveal a grade 2 endometriod carcinoma confined to the uterine fundus. She has uncontrolled diabetes and hypertension and her BMI is 35 kg/m^2.

    What is the most appropriate next step in the management?

A. Perform a MRI scan

B. Perform total hysterectomy and bilateral salpingo-oophorectomy.

C. Perform total hysterectomy, bilateral salpingo-oophorectomy, pelvic and para-aortic lymph node dissection.

D. Preoperative radiotherapy followed by total hysterectomy and bilateral salpingo-oophorectomy.

E. Treat with a high dose of progestogens.

5. A 56-year-old woman presents with postmenopausal bleeding. Hysteroscopy and biopsy reveal an endometrial carcinoma confined to the uterine fundus. Histology reveals a grade 1 endometriod carcinoma. MRI scan reveals less than 50% myometrial involvement.

What is the most appropriate treatment?

A. Piver type three extended hysterectomy.

B. Preoperative radiotherapy followed by total hysterectomy and bilateral salpingo-oophorectomy.

C. Total hysterectomy and bilateral salpingo-oophorectomy.

D. Total hysterectomy, bilateral salpingo-oophorectomy and pelvic lymph node dissection.

E. Total hysterectomy, bilateral salpingo-oophorectomy, pelvic and para-aortic lymph node dissection.

6. A 56-year-old woman presents with postmenopausal bleeding. Hysteroscopy and biopsy reveal an endometrial carcinoma confined to the uterine fundus. Histology reveals a grade two clear cell carcinoma. MRI scan reveals less than 50% myometrial invasion.

What is the most appropriate treatment?

A. Piver type 3 hysterectomy.

B. Preoperative radiotherapy followed by total hysterectomy and bilateral salpingo-oophorectomy.

C. Total hysterectomy and bilateral salpingo-oophorectomy.

D. Total hysterectomy, bilateral salpingo-oophorectomy and pelvic lymph node dissection.

E. Total hysterectomy, bilateral salpingo-oophorectomy, pelvic and para-aortic lymph node dissection.

7. A 60-year-old woman presents with post-menopausal bleeding. A diagnosis of a grade 2 endometrioid carcinoma confined to the fundus and invading more than 50% of the myometrium is made.

What is the most appropriate treatment?

A. Piver type three extended hysterectomy.

B. Preoperative chemotherapy followed by total hysterectomy and bilateral salpingo-oophorectomy.

C. Preoperative radiotherapy followed by total hysterectomy and bilateral salpingo-oophorectomy.

D. Total hysterectomy and bilateral salpingo-oophorectomy.

E. Total hysterectomy, bilateral salpingo-oophorectomy, pelvic and para-aortic lymph node dissection.

8. A 63-year-old woman with type 2 diabetes mellitus complains of 2 episodes of mild vaginal bleeding over the past 3 months. There is no history of vaginal discharge. Her past medical history is significant for anxiety disorders, depression, hypertension and gout. Her BMI is 35 kg/m^2.

What is the most likely cause for her symptoms?

A. Cervical carcinoma

B. Endometrial carcinoma

C. Ovarian carcinoma

D. Vaginal cancer

E. Vulvar cancer

9. A 63-year-old woman with type 2 diabetes mellitus complains of 2 episodes of mild vaginal bleeding over the past 3 months. There is no history of vaginal

discharge. Her past medical history is significant for anxiety disorders, depression, hypertension and gout. Her BMI is 30 kg/m². Abdominal vaginal and speculum examinations are normal.

What is the most appropriate step to arrive at a diagnosis ?

A. Cervical cytology.

B. Hysterectomy and bilateral salpingo-oophorectomy.

C. Hysteroscopy and biopsy.

D. Pipelle aspiration.

E. Transvaginal ultrasound scan.

ANSWERS AND EXPLANATIONS

Q. 1 (E), Q. 2 (B) and Q. 3 (B)

Explanation for questions 1, 2 and 3

Transvaginal ultrasound scanning is the first investigation which should be performed in a woman who presents with peri or postmenopausal bleeding. An endometrial thickness of less than 4 mm has a negative predictive value for endometrial carcinoma and the patient can be kept under observation. A repeat scan should be performed in 3 months. If the endometrial thickness is more than 4 mm, endometrial sampling is necessary. Even if the thickening is uniform, because the endometrium is thin in a postmenopausal woman and incidence of cancer is high, hysteroscopy and biopsy is a better option than pipelle aspiration. Dilatation and curettage and fractional curettage are of limited value because an early lesion can be missed. If there is focal thickening hysteroscopy is essential as direct visualization is necessary and the biopsy should be taken from the thickened area.

Q. 4 (A)

A MRI scan should be performed first to assess the spread of the tumour, in order to plan the best surgical procedure. Since this patient is obese and has co-morbidities increasing the operative risk, it is even more important to determine the extent of the surgical procedure according to the extent of the disease. If the tumour has not infiltrated more than 50% of the myometrium and the lymph nodes appear to be normal in the preoperative assessment, laparoscopic hysterectomy and BSO without lymph node dissection would be the best option. If higher risk features are found at surgery or on histopathological examination, adjuvant radiotherapy may be considered in conjunction with an oncologist. Laparoscopy is preferred in obese women because of the lower incidence of wound infection and shorter hospital stay. If a laparotomy is performed, it is best combined with an abdominoplasty.

Q 5 (C)

This woman falls into the low risk category as she has a stage IA G1, endometriod type carcinoma. Therefore, total abdominal hysterectomy and BSO is the best treatment option. Peritoneal washings are taken for cytology, lymph nodes are palpated and suspicious nodes are sampled. If higher risk features are found at surgery or on histopathological examination, adjuvant radiotherapy may be considered in conjunction with an oncologist.

Q. 6 (E)

Even though this woman has a stage I A G2 endometrial carcinoma she falls into the high risk category as she has a clear cell carcinoma. Therefore, the best management option is total hysterectomy, bilateral salpingo-oophorectomy, pelvic and para-aortic lymph node dissection.

Q. 7 (E)

This woman has a stage IB endometrial carcinoma. Therefore, the best management option is total hysterectomy, bilateral salpingo-oophorectomy, pelvic and para–aortic lymph node dissection.

Q. 8 (B) and Q. 9 (C)

Explanation for questions 8 and 9

This woman most probably has endometrial carcinoma because she has the following risk factors.

Older age

Diabetes mellitus

Hypertension

Gout

Depression

Obesity

She has no risk factors for the other cancers. Examination findings are normal, further indicating the possibility of endometrial cancer. The next step in the management is to perform a transvaginal ultrasound scan to assess the endometrial thickness. However, hysteroscopy is the most appropriate test to arrive at a diagnosis. It should be performed even if the TVUS is normal, because she is at high risk of endometrial carcinoma. Cervical cytology should be done if it has not been performed within the last 3 years.

REFERENCES

- J.L. Benedet, H. Bender, H. Jones III, H.Y.S. Ngan, S. Pecorelli. Staging classifications and clinical practice guidelines of gynaecologic cancers—FIGO Committee on Gynaecologic Oncology.
- Endometrial Hyperplasia, Management of Green-top Guideline No. 67, Published: 26/02/2016.

17

Utero-vaginal Prolapse

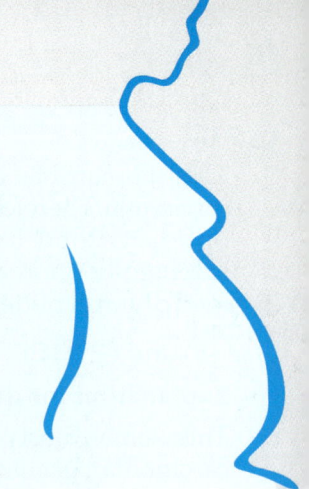

AETIOLOGY

- Repeated childbirth.
  - Stretching and tearing of the endopelvic fascia, levator ani muscles and muscles of the perineal body cause pelvic floor defects.
  - Partial pudendal and perineal neuropathies can be caused by labour. Impaired nerve transmission to the muscles of the pelvic floor may result in decreased tone, causing further sagging and stretching.
- Genital atrophy due to low oestrogen levels at menopause.
- Connective tissue abnormalities.
- Increased intra-abdominal pressure.
  - Pelvic tumours
  - Chronic cough
- Chronic constipation.
- Obesity.
- Neurological disorders.
  - Sacral nerve disorders
  - Diabetic neuropathy

There are three levels of pelvic support for the vagina and the cervix.

- Level 1 supports
  - Uterosacral ligaments and the transverse ligaments (Mackenrodt ligaments) supporting the cervix and upper vagina. Defects arising at this level lead to uterine descent or vault descent.
- Level 2 supports
  - Pubocervical fascia and rectovaginal fascia, supporting the anterior and posterior vaginal walls, by attaching to the arcus tendineus. Defects at this level lead to anterior and posterior vaginal wall prolapse.
- Level 3 supports
  - Consist of the direct attachment of the distal part of vagina to the pubic bone anteriorly and the perineal body posteriorly. Levator ani muscles form the pelvic diaphragm which plays a major role at this level.

EXAMINATION AND STAGING

Assessment of the prolapse must be done with these anatomical supports in mind. Patient is examined in the lithotomy position using a Sim's speculum. The standing position can be used to confirm the results.

Stage I	Descent of the uterus to any point in the vagina up to 1 cm proximal to the hymen
Stage II	Descent from 1 cm proximal to the hymen, to the hymen, or up to 1 cm distal to the hymen
Stage III	Descent beyond 1 cm distal to the hymen
Stage IV	Total uterine prolapse or uterine procidentia

COMPONENTS OF PROLAPSE

- Uterine descent
- Descent of the anterior vaginal wall with the underlying bladder—cystocele
- Descent of the posterior vaginal wall with the underlying rectum—rectocele
- Apical prolapse—enterocele

SYMPTOMS

- Lump at vulva, feeling of fullness in the vagina, dragging sensation in the perineum, difficulty in sexual intercourse, dyspareunia and backache.

Urinary Symptoms

- Difficulty to initiate voiding of urine, feeling of incomplete voiding and the need to digitate, stress incontinence, urgency and recurrent urinary tract infection.

Bowel Symptoms

- Difficulty in emptying the bowel, the need to digitate, feeling of incomplete emptying and soiling.

Decubitus Ulcers

- These are formed in the most dependant area of the prolapse round the cervix, due to poor nutrition caused by venous congestion.
- They cause bleeding and discharge.
- Infection and bleeding can occur if surgery is performed in the presence of decubitus ulcers.
- The prolapse should be kept reduced with a pessary to cause healing of ulcers. Oestrogen cream may facilitate healing in postmenopausal women.

Treatment

- Conservative treatment
  - Weight loss
  - Avoid lifting heavy weights
  - Avoid constipation
  - Pelvic floor exercises

- Insertion of a pessary is the first line treatment,
  - during pregnancy and puerperium,
  - if the woman wishes to complete the family soon,
  - if there is a serious uncorrectable medical problem,
  - to heal a decubitus ulcer prior to surgery,
  - if the woman refuses surgery.

Pessaries can alleviate most of the symptoms of prolapse including voiding symptoms, urgency-related symptoms, bowel symptoms and sexual difficulties, but not stress incontinence.

Minor complications from pessary use include bleeding, discomfort and discharge, which may be offensive. Major complications such as incarceration and vaginal fistulae are rare and are often due to neglected pessaries. Therefore, it is important to change pessaries regularly once in 3–6 months.

SURGERY

Vaginal Hysterectomy and Repair

- It is the first line treatment for women who do not wish to preserve their fertility.
- Vaginal hysterectomy should be combined with anterior (cystocele repair), posterior (rectocele repair) and apical repair. (enterocele and vault repair).

Uterus Preserving Surgical Procedures

- Contraindications for uterine preservation include abnormal uterine bleeding, cervical dysplasia and presence of fibroids.
- Uterine preservation is difficult in the presence of 4th degree prolapse.
- Uterine preservation is indicated only if the woman wishes to preserve her fertility.

Manchester Repair

- This procedure is recommended for patients with elongation of the cervix. However, difficulties may occur in future pregnancies due to cervical incompetence and cervical stenosis.

Sacrohysteropexy

- Can be done by the vaginal, abdominal or laparoscopic routes

- Restores and reinforces uterine support by suspending the uterus from the sacral promontory using type 1 polypropylene mesh.
- Restores vaginal length. Restoration of apical support results in a reduction in the anterior prolapse and enterocele.

QUESTIONS

1. A 70-year-old otherwise healthy woman complains of urgency incontinence. On examination there is no evidence of utero-vaginal prolapse. The ultrasound scan, urine full report and fasting blood sugar are within normal limits.

   What is the best management option?
   A. Bladder training.
   B. Insertion of a transobturator tension free vaginal tape.
   C. Low dose nalidixic acid for three months.
   D. Pelvic floor exercises.
   E. Treatment with oxybutinon.

2. A 35-year-old woman who has delivered her third baby two months ago complains of urgency incontinence. On examination there is no evidence of utero-vaginal prolapse. The ultrasound scan, urine full report and fasting blood sugar are within normal limits.

   What is the best management option?
   A. Bladder training.
   B. Insertion of a *trans* obturator tension free vaginal tape.
   C. Low dose nalidixic acid for three months.
   D. Pelvic floor exercises.
   E. Treatment with oxybutinon.

3. A 65-year-old patient with diabetes mellitus and hypertension has a 3rd degree utero-vaginal prolapse. She gives a history of several episodes of urinary retention which needed catheterization at the local hospital.

   What is the best management option?
   A. Anterior and posterior repair.
   B. Insertion of a polyvinyl ring pessary.
   C. Manchester repair.
   D. Vaginal hysterectomy.
   E. Vaginal hysterectomy and repair.

4. A 65-year-old patient has a 3rd degree utero-vaginal prolapse with a large decubitus ulcer. She gives a history of several episodes of urinary retention which needed catheterization at the local hospital.

   What is the next step in the management of this patient?
   A. Insertion of a polyvinyl ring pessary and application of oestrogen cream
   B. Manchester repair
   C. Vaginal hysterectomy and repair
   D. Anterior and posterior repair
   E. Daily application of betadine cream and oestrogen cream

5. A 33-year-old woman with two children has a second degree utero-vaginal prolapse with a cystocele and rectocele. She wishes to conceive soon to complete her family.

   What is the best management option?
   A. Anterior and posterior repair
   B. Insertion of a pessary
   C. Manchester repair
   D. Pelvic floor exercises
   E. Sacrohysteropexy

6. **A 35-year-old woman with two children has a second degree utero-vaginal prolapse with a cystocele, rectocele and an enterocele. She does not wish to conceive soon but wishes to retain her fertility.**

   What is the best management option?

   A. Anterior and posterior repair

   B. Insertion of a pessary

   C. Manchester repair

   D. Pelvic floor exercises

   E. Sacrohysteropexy

7. **A 60-year-old otherwise healthy woman without any other uterine pathology has a first degree utero-vaginal prolapse with a cystocele.**

   What is the best management option?

   A. Insertion of a pessary

   B. Manchester repair

   C. Pelvic floor exercises

   D. Sacrohysteropexy

   E. Vaginal hysterectomy and repair

ANSWERS AND EXPLANATIONS

Q. 1 (E)

Even though bladder training is the first line treatment option, it may not be easy to do so in a 70-year-old woman, whose bladder and pelvic floor musculature may be weak. Therefore, the best treatment option is to commence oxybutinon 5 mg twice or thrice daily. This treatment can be combined with bladder training to obtain long-term relief. Oxybutynin is an anticholinergic drug which causes direct smooth muscle relaxation of the urinary bladder and has local anaesthetic properties. It is contraindicated in those with cardiac disease, liver disease, glaucoma, myasthenia gravis and porphyria. Adverse effects include blurred vision, dry mouth, heart palpitations, drowsiness, and facial flushing. Darifenacin, solifenacin, and trospium have shown efficacy comparable to that of oxybutynin and with less adverse effects.

Q. 2 (A)

A vesical calculus, urinary tract infection and diabetes mellitus should be first excluded in those with urgency.

First line therapy for urinary urgency is bladder training which can be combined with drug therapy if required. Since this woman is young and has delivered a baby two months ago bladder training is the first line treatment option. She should be advised to hold her urine for longer periods each day.

Q. 3 (E)

Since this woman has a third degree utero-vaginal prolapse the best management option is vaginal hysterectomy and repair. Vaginal hysterectomy should be combined with anterior (cystocele repair), posterior (rectocele repair) and apical repair (enterocele repair), to obtain a complete cure and to prevent recurrence. There is no indication for pessary treatment, as she has no contraindications for surgery, which provides a definitive cure. Diabetes mellitus and hypertension should be controlled prior to performing surgery. Anterior and posterior repair will not cure her symptoms as she has an uterine prolapse as well.

Q. 4 (A)

This woman needs a vaginal hysterectomy and repair as she has a third degree utero-vaginal prolapse, but bleeding and infection can occur if surgery is performed in the presence of a decubitus ulcer. Therefore, the first step in the management is to heal the ulcer. Decubitus ulcers occur in the most dependant part of the prolapse, due to venous congestion resulting in tissue oedema and poor nutrition. Therefore, the first step in the management is to keep the prolapse reduced by inserting a pessary. Healing can be expedited by application of iodine or oestrogen cream in a postmenopausal woman. The prolapse can also be reduced with a tampon or pack soaked in betadine. However, these are less convenient as they have to be changed daily.

Q. 5 (B)

Q. 6 (E)

If a woman who has an utero-vaginal prolapse wishes to conceive soon, the best management option is to insert a pessary. Surgery could be performed about 1 year after the delivery.

If a woman who does not wish to conceive soon wishes to preserve her fertility the best option is sacrohysteropexy which can be performed by laparoscopy or through an abdominal incision. Manchester operation is also an option but cervical stenosis and cervical incompetence can occur during a future pregnancy.

Q. 7 (D)

Since this woman has a first degree uterine prolapse and a cystocoele only, without any other uterine pathology, sacrohysteropexy is a better option than vaginal hysterectomy, which is a more major procedure.